Fleeting
(For Mom)
Fleeting memories.
Too fleeting to hold.
Too precious to let go.

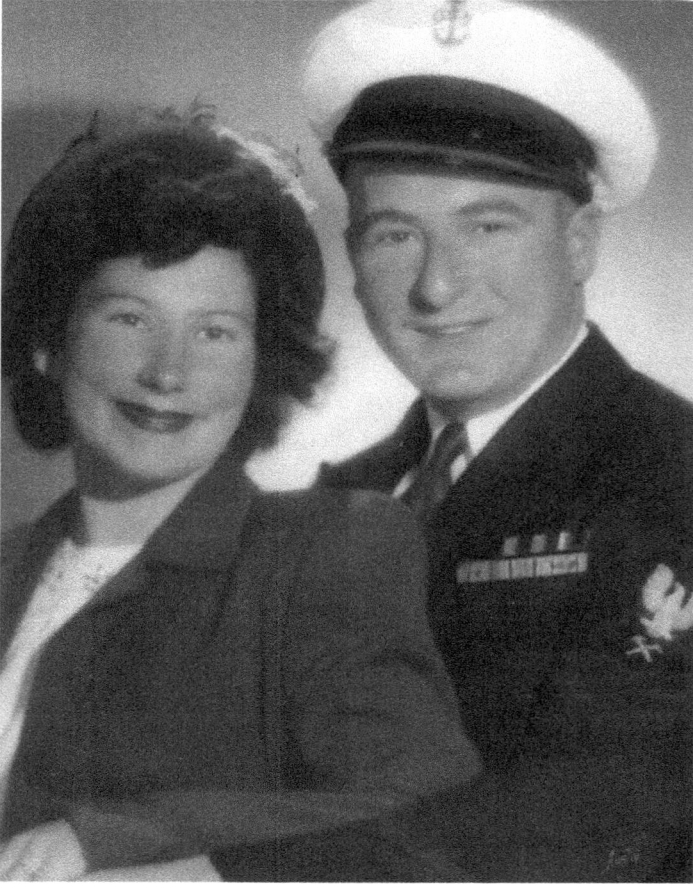

Velva & Cecil Jones

If I Forget

A Caregiver's Memories

Judy Jones

AVAILABLE AT AMAZON.COM

ISBN - 10: 061543343X

ISBN-13: 978-0615433431

(Dunbar-Jones Publishing)

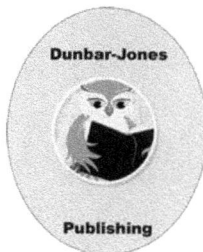

DEDICATION

If I Forget honors the memory of my beloved grandmother, Mattie Dunbar; my mother, Velva Dunbar Jones; and my aunts, Hazel and Marjorie, who all lived and died with dementia.

If I Forget is dedicated to loving caregivers such as my father, Cecil Jones, who stood fast at my mother's side until his last exhausted breath.

ACKNOWLEDGMENTS

Many family members and friends are responsible for this book reaching print, and I thank them all. Two very dear friends stand out for spending many hours editing the final product.

Retired Col. Fred Peck, USMC, is a friend, former supervisor, an award-winning journalist and a publisher. Fred, co-owner of Bolder Voices Inc., not only offered proofing expertise; he pointed me in a direction that made this book complete.

Sonja Kosler is an award-winning poet and storyteller. We have been friends through many phases of our lives. Sonja's mentorship and her precision in editing kept this story flowing smoothly. Her encouraging words, kept me going. Sonja also reminded me my first edition need not be perfection. That's what subsequent editions are for. If not for that reminder, I would still be editing, proofing and rewriting.

I also want to thank Rodney Deutschmann of the San Diego In Focus Learning Center for the beautiful cover photo of my mother and me. Thank you Fred, Sonja, my family and my friends for all the kind words and gentle encouragement from the first word to the last.

Table of Contents

VALENTINE'S DAY 1999

HEARTS BREAK

"Do you have to leave so soon?"

I looked into Dad's pleading eyes as I was about to end our weekly Sunday visit. There was something there I had never before seen. Was it loneliness? Was it weariness from taking care of Mom? It was something I could not quite read.

He never lets anyone help him. He couldn't help but be exhausted. Did I see fear? I had never seen fear on Dad's face. He was fearless. He was my rock, my strength. He could not be afraid. I did not allow that thought to linger in my mind.

As I started to say goodbye, I saw something else there in his face, in his posture. This, too, was something I had never seen. My mind was racing through the things I had to do today. It was Valentine's Day.

I glanced at the photo I was holding. It was taken that morning at Dad's favorite buffet, where we enjoyed our weekly breakfast. Mom and

Daddy sat under an arch of red, pink and white balloons. A Valentine's Day place of honor for those married more than 50 years.

There it was – *that look*. It was the *look* in his eyes I now see. Odd, I didn't notice *that look* when they took the photo.

"Well, sure, I can stay longer," I gave in. His face brightened, but there was still that disturbing look in his eyes.

"I want to show you something," he said, slowly hobbling into the family room, his body tired and pain-filled from a lifetime of hard labor, broken bones and a broken heart.

I followed and tried to help him wrestle his telescope from the corner, but he gently pushed me away.

"It's OK kid. I got it," he said gruffly as he struggled to drag it outside.

I am so glad I gave him that telescope. He had a ball with it. He couldn't get out much because Mom could not be left alone and was difficult to control on outings. So, it gave him something to do other than sit in front of the TV.

I got the idea for the telescope when Dad was trying to view the 1997 Hale-Bopp comet through his binoculars. The comet held a special fascination for him. In my lifetime, I had never known the heavens to intrigue him so, other than to comment, "how pretty the stars are tonight."

We set the telescope up together on the patio. From their hilltop home, there was nearly a 360-degree view. He fiddled with the knobs as he looked through the viewer. He seemed frustrated.

"Mmmm, why are we setting up the telescope on this bright sunny day? We sure won't see anything in the sky," I thought to myself. "Oh, well, humor him Judy."

"God damn it all to Hell," he growled as he tried to adjust the viewer. "Can you look through this bastard and focus on the hill across the valley?"

I am no telescope guru, but I managed to zero in on the hilltop and could clearly see what I could not before – a house and all its happenings. I looked at Dad. His mischievous twinkle had returned to his eyes, almost covering that other look. The look I could not describe. The look that was so disconcerting.

"Dad, are you becoming a peeping Tom in your old age?" I joked. "I got you this to watch the stars, not your neighbors."

"Oh yeah, you should see the goings-on in the neighborhood," he laughed his big deep roar of a laugh, a little weaker than normal. I love his laugh. You can't help but feel good when you hear it. And, you can certainly hear it. When I was little, if I lost track of him, all I had to do was listen for this big laugh.

"I just want to see how far away you can get on this God damned thing. Hell, my old eyes, just can't God damn focus it in."

There it is, the eyes thing again. Even he was talking about his old eyes. I was so glad I stayed. He was having so much fun with this.

Mom was inside napping, giving us some father-daughter time away from her increasingly demented mind. It had been a long while since we could spend time like this together.

It seemed harsh, and I felt guilty for thinking this, but given Mom's descent into Alzheimer's Hell, I looked forward to when God finally allowed her to reclaim her soul and her dignity in Heaven.

Maybe Dad and I can fix this old place up and even take a road trip back home to Iowa. As a Daddy's girl who spent every possible minute by his side, it has been a difficult journey for us. We had lost Mom to Alzheimer's and, with it, our companionship.

"Well, Daddy, I really do have to go now, I have someone expecting me this afternoon," I told him as we hugged.

He seemed frailer. His body had not changed in size, but his strength was gone, zapped, I suppose, by the endless hours of taking care of Mom. When my condo sale goes through, I'll put everything in storage and move in to help him, whether he objects or not. He cannot continue carrying this burden alone.

Our hug lasted longer than usual. He was never much of a hugger. Neither am I, for that matter. Today, Dad did not want to let go. I wished I didn't have other plans. I should have stayed there, I thought regretfully.

"You'd better get going Yogi," he said, as he released his hold, and called me by the pet name he gave me with when I was a child.

As I pulled out of the driveway, I saw him at the top of the patio stairs. He watched me. I saw him in my rearview mirror, still there. He had never done that before. A horrible dreading welled up from deep inside. It's that dreading I get before tragedy strikes. I'm not sure I can describe the feeling. It comes from the pit of my stomach, takes over my whole being and whirls me into a tailspin that ends only when this portent manifests. Until then, an opaque curtain of dread clouds my mind.

I'M VELVA DUNBAR – PART I

HOO, WHO?

"Hoo?" hooted the owl outside the window, breaking the silence of the summer night.

"Velva Dunbar," the toddler responded, looking outside to see who was talking to her.

"Hoo, hoo?" the owl persisted.

"I'm Velva Dunbar," the toddler repeated.

"Hoo?" again the owl.

"I tells ya, I'm Velva Dunbar!"

Velva La Verne Dunbar was the first born of Mattie Landreth Dunbar and Clinton Dunbar. She came into this world in St. James Illinois, a speck of a town so small you can't find it on maps.

St. James barely exists today. In Mom's day, the small town boasted a train station, store, school and churches.

Church life formed the community identity. Most prominent, at least in Mom's tales, were the extremely conservative Free Methodists, Seventh Day Adventists and Disciples of Christ. It was the latter church that Mom attended with her grandmother, divorcee Caroline Dunbar, who rocked the community when she gave her abusive husband, John, the boot. John Dunbar was a town constable who was known for his Tennessee walker horses. He had to take some time off from his constable duties to serve jail sentences for failure to provide financial support to his ex-wife.

"He had piercing blue eyes and dark demeanor that struck fear in those who encountered him," his grandson Roy Dunbar recalled.

The Dunbars were a poor but proud family, even before the Great Depression. Clint was among third-generation Scottish-Americans from the Dunbar clan, which reportedly immigrated to the United States with a great deal of money that the not-so-thrifty Dunbar brothers squandered.

As poor as the Dunbars were at the time, they must have seemed wealthy to young Mattie Landreth, whose parents sent her into servitude at about 12 years old to help support her 10 brothers and sisters. It was easy to see why she was smitten with the handsome, funny, sweet-talking Clint Dunbar.

Clint tried to farm the poor soil in St. James. He was not raised a farmer, had only a few acres and knew little of the farming business – not a recipe for success.

When he was a young single man, Clint worked for the Illinois Central Railway, with runs from Chicago to New Orleans. He was fired after he and a co-worker took a joy ride down the railroad tracks on a company handcart to see some girls. After his marriage to Mattie, and quickly having a family to support, he wrote an eloquent letter to the head of the railroad company asking for reinstatement.

"I was young and brash," Clint wrote. *"I am sorry my actions. Now, I am married with a family. If you reinstate me, I will prove to be a valuable and responsible employee."*

Clint got his job back as a brakeman, then was promoted to conductor. He retired from the railroad many years later.

"Our house was just off the railroad tracks," Velva would tell her children. "He had a special whistle that the engineer would blow when the train passed through St. James. That way we knew it was him."

The Dunbar girls loved when Clint was home. He was the kind of dad who got down on his hands and knees, giving them all pony rides and having tickling matches. But, Clint was gone a lot, and rumor has it he had a girl at every whistle stop. He would be home long enough to produce another child and leave a little money for Mattie – very little money.

"Mom, worked so hard to earn money growing and selling produce, eggs, her hand-woven rugs – whatever she could – to keep food on the table," Velva remembered. "As soon as us kids were old enough, she took us along to pick strawberries in the local fields. It was backbreaking even for us youngin's. I remember one Christmas, when Dad left us with no money. I remember my mom crying because all she had to put in our stockings was one orange each."

Those whistle stops in St. James added Hazel, Marjorie, Evelyn and Roy to the community's Dunbar population count. In between were miscarriages.

"I was looking through Mom's papers one day and found a letter she had written to the Lady's Home Journal," Velva said. "She begged them to print information on how to stop having so many children. She was so tired and in such poor health .... It was heartbreaking."

When Velva was a teenager, her mom miscarried after being pushed down the stairs by Clint. A fight ensued between Velva and her father – a fight that fractured a once strong bond between father and daughter. Velva was sent away after that to live with her Uncle Roy Landreth and his wife in Chicago. Roy was an executive running the Chicago railroad yard – probably the reason his sister's new husband was given back his job. Velva vowed she would never put up with a man physically abusing her. She also vowed never to have children. She wanted a career as a schoolteacher.

While living in Chicago, Velva grew to love big city life. She loved the excitement, the crowds, the theater, museums and zoo. Her Uncle Roy and his wife were childless, so they showered Velva with attention. It was with great reluctance that she returned home to help her mother.

Things were not always strained between Velva and her dad. As a child, she spent every second with him when he was home. She left the cooking and sewing to her sisters. She had no interest in "womanly" things. Instead, she and Clint would hit the woods for hunting, or the local ponds for fishing. She learned her love of outdoors through Clint.

The locals, however, were not impressed with her unruly tomboy ways.

"I loved riding horses, and my Grandpa Dunbar had beautiful horses," Velva said. "One hot summer day, a friend and I cutoff our dad's Levis into short-shorts, borrowed one of Grandpa's horses and rode into town bareback. The local preachers were up in arms over this joy ride by the short-short clad girls. Sermons were preached that Sunday about the corruption of the youth of the day."

If not impressed by her notorious ride, townsfolk were impressed in other ways. St. James kids were educated in an all-grades, one-room school that went only to the 11th grade. Velva was a straight "A" student. She also was one of the school's best athletes, playing baseball and basketball right alongside the boys. If there had been football, she would have been on that team, too.

"I wasn't much to look at," Velva said. "I was skinny. No figure at all. I had a face full of freckles and the kids teased me unmercifully. I also was painfully shy."

Velva did draw the attention of one boy, who tried to attack her sexually by ambushing her on the way home from school. She left him bruised, bleeding, and blaming Velva for encouraging the attack.

"I had a pretty bad temper back then," she said. "I learned to control it after I almost killed one of my sisters. We did not have disposable sanitary napkins. We used rags. Us girls, each had only two – one to use, one to wash. Hazel got her period, but was too embarrassed to tell anyone. Instead, she took my rags, soiled them and then hid them under the bed.

"Mom found them and I got in trouble for not cleaning my rags. I was so furious at Hazel that I jumped on her, pushed her to the floor and started banging her head until she almost lost consciousness. I almost killed by sister. I vowed that day to never let myself get that angry again."

As an adult, Velva slipped up during one of many arguments with her second husband Chuck. This particular fight, out of frustration, she hurled a cast iron skillet at him. He ducked, and the kitchen wall had a permanent indent. Never argue with a woman in the kitchen. She never asked Chuck to repair it, and he never offered. I think they left it there as a reminder never to get that angry again.

Velva channeled her passions away from anger and to political activism, working on numerous campaigns and serving as the treasurer of the San Diego Democratic Central Committee. Her love of politics she inherited from her dad. Besides railway work and womanizing, Clint was an active Mason, and a tireless campaigner in local and state politics for the Democratic Party. At one point in the pre-Depression era, he joined the Socialist Party. He soon became disenchanted with the Socialists and went back to the Democrats.

"No matter what else he was, no matter how much he failed his family in so many ways, Dad had respect in the community as both a vital, active member, and also as an honest man who was true to his word and paid his debts," Velva often said.

These were values Velva lived by and passed on to her children and grandchildren.

FEBRUARY 18, 1999

THE PHONE CALL

"Hi Mom, where's Daddy?"

"Oh, he's out in the yard working like always. I tried getting him to come in, but you know that man is pig headed. He'll be in later," Mom says sounding abnormally normal.

How unusual my usual phone call just turned. I call home to Dad every Thursday. Mom stopped answering the phone a few years ago; it was too confusing for her. Part of me wants to believe she has recovered from Alzheimer's. But, I know there is no recovery.

She does have lucid moments. Sometimes it's minutes; sometimes it's hours. You just never know. They get fewer and shorter as time goes on.

"I'll be there on Sunday for our visit," I tell her, pushing down that deep dreading rising up from my gut.

Something is not right. Dad has not been able to do yard work for a long time. Mom no longer answers the phone.

"What is happening? I'm sure things are fine," I assure myself.

"The YANA folks will be out to see them today. They'll let me know if something is wrong."

I'm sure glad I signed Mom and Dad up with the Sheriff's Department to have weekly visits and phone calls from the senior volunteers' YANA (You Are Not Alone). It gives Dad a midweek break from nonsensical conversations with Mom and gives me some peace of mind that they are OK. Dad is funny about those YANA people.

"We don't need no sons-a-bitchin' old farts comin' 'round checkin' up on us," he told me when I suggested it.

As usual, I ignored his objections.

I know by his comments after their visits that he is grateful. He'll never admit it, though. He never admits anything. Not even how hard Mom's Alzheimer's is on him.

It's getting worse. We all were devastated when she was diagnosed with Alzheimer's. She has never accepted the diagnosis. It had been her great fear that she would lose herself to dementia, as did her mother.

"See, the doctor told me after those tests that I'm smart," Mom protested, after Alzheimer's screening confirmed all our fears. "So I obviously can't have Alzheimer's."

We started losing Mom to Alzheimer's about 20 years ago, when she was in her 60s. We didn't know it at the time. We thought it was just normal aging. It did stick in the back of our minds as she became more forgetful and was having difficulty using words correctly.

Two of mom's sisters and Grandma Dunbar, her mom, had Alzheimer's or dementia. We were not unfamiliar with the symptoms. But we did not want to acknowledge the possibility.

My sister, brother, Daddy and I talked about the possibility of Alzheimer's or maybe small strokes. Mom would not acknowledge any problems, however, even after the diagnosis of this always fatal disease.

The odds don't look good for my sister, Carolyn, and me. Our brother, Danny, died four months ago, his body ravaged by years of smoking, so he needs not worry about Alzheimer's. Maybe that is why he would not give up smoking, even after a heart bypass. Dying with heart and lung disease was easier than the thought of losing who you are to dementia.

One of the first telling signs of Mom's disease appeared with a memory lapse as she said grace over Thanksgiving dinner. She had never said grace before. Dad or another male relative would do that honor. She gave this long rambling grace, and then went around the table God blessing everyone. She came to Roland, my then-husband, and stopped. She looked over at him and said, "I'm sorry, what is your name? Not as if she had a momentary lapse, but as if he were a stranger at the table. We all looked at each other, knowing this was not a good sign.

By Easter, she plunged further into that crazy Alzheimer's world. I invited family and friends for my annual Easter brunch.

She and Daddy were on their weekly grocery-shopping trip a few days before Easter. Mom began looking for a turkey for the "Thanksgiving dinner. "

This was not just a slip of saying Thanksgiving instead of Easter. This was a full-on insistence that it was Thanksgiving, and she needed to purchase a turkey for the dinner. She was very irritated at Dad. He called me that evening so I could convince her that it was Easter, and I was fixing a brunch.

"Mom, it's not Thanksgiving. It's Easter. I'm making Easter brunch. You don't need to do anything," I explained over and over and over.

"Well, if you say so, then I guess it must be," she finally gave in.

We were losing her. As time went on, things went downhill, which is the only direction Alzheimer's takes. There were the frightened phone calls from Mom telling me there was a strange man in the house. There were the anguished calls from Dad, because Mom insisted he was not her husband, and she was going to call the police. Her husband, she said, was Carson, a man who in reality she had married and divorced more than 60 years ago.

Months before, Dad had to stop going to the local American Legion hall with Mom. The hall holds cheap weekly dinners and breakfasts. The food, the bar with cheap drinks and the camaraderie gave Dad a good respite – a sense of sanity in the midst of insanity.

Mom began flirting and making moves on a bartender there – a man in his 40s. This was so out of character for this usually modest woman. It became so uncomfortable for everyone that Dad decided it was best they no longer go to the hall. He wouldn't – actually couldn't – leave her alone at home, so this was a fatal blow to his last shred of male friendship.

Alzheimer's shackled Mom. It imprisoned Dad.

"Anytime you see Jonesy, you will see Velva. He never leaves her side," a local once told me.

Two years ago, after much pleading, Dad let me take Mom shopping and to lunch, like we used to do. I saw that she badly needed some new clothing, and Dad needed a break. Turned out Mom needed one, too.

"Oh boy, am I ever glad to get out of there and away from that man. He's always hangin' around," Mom said in a hushed, conspiratorial tone as she buckled up her seatbelt. I had to chuckle.

I figured Dad would go to the Legion Hall to visit old friends and have a beer or two. But, no. He stayed home and fretted the whole time. When we got back, I found him pacing the property, just the way he used to do when Carolyn or I went out on a date. I told him we had a great time, and there were no problems.

"Mom enjoyed herself. It was good for her to get out with me," I said. "See, she is fine."

"Yeah, but she's all wored out now and will be battier than a God damned bat later. You just don't know," he grumbled with a hint of dread in his voice.

I pooh-poohed him. But, he never let me take her anywhere again. He was right. I didn't know. He didn't let me or anyone know the reality of his life.

I wish I lived closer so I could have seen them daily during past years. I could have held them when they faced these horrible moments. I could have carried some of Dad's burden. I commend him for taking such good care of Mom all those years. This man, hardened by Depression era farm life, surviving the sinking of his ship in World War II, followed by years of hard labor on construction sites, had become the homemaker, the caregiver. Sort of ironic. Sort of sad.

He calls me to get advice on cooking. He was so proud when he mastered stuffed peppers. He does the shopping, the finances, the laundry and the house cleaning. Well, he tries with the house cleaning. But as his back, leg and hand pain worsens, his ability to keep the house clean dwindles. I've tried several times to spend the day cleaning, only to have him insist I stop so we could have lunch, or dinner or just sit and visit.

"God damn it, Yogi, I don't want you over here cleaning," he would growl. "I want you to come to visit with us. The house can go plum to God damned hell."

Today is different. Mom answered the phone and Dad, I'm told, is working in the yard. That's how it used to be. But that's not how it is, now. Except today ....

Maybe I should rush out there now. Take off from work tomorrow.

"Don't worry Judy," I tell myself, "YANA will be coming by soon. If something is wrong, they'll call. I hope."

I'M VELVA DUNBAR – PART II

The Old Chief and the Divorcee

Cecil C. Jones and Velva Dunbar married Nov. 3, 1946 after a brief and unusual courtship. Velva was a divorcee working many jobs to support her two children. Her ex-husband was abusive, and according to family members a drunk. Velva was reluctant to speak ill of the father of her son and daughter, Danny and Carolyn. Danny made a rough start in this world. He was born breach and nearly died.

"There were no hospitals, so he was born at home. I had no anesthesia," Velva mentioned whenever one of her children was giving birth. "He was blue when he was born. I thought he was dead."

Danny proved to be a sickly child for his first few years. But with a mother's love and nurturing he reached adulthood-- a thin but healthy 6 feet at the time he entered the Marine Corps. He swore he was 6'1" when he went to boot camp, but the drill instructors beat him down to 6 feet by the time he graduated.

Velva tried to raise Danny to respect and treat others with kindness.

"I used to send him to school with really cute caps," Velva recalled. "Every day, he would come home without his cap. When I asked him about it he would say someone liked it, so he gave it to them. His teacher told me that the boys at school were stealing his caps. When I asked him about why he let them steal his caps he told me because I had taught him not to fight. I was forced to face the truth that sometimes you just have to fight. I told him he needed to stand up to the bullies. He did and he never had another cap stolen – or anything else for that matter."

Velva moved to San Diego with her then-husband, Roy Carson, in the early 1940s from Southern Illinois. In 1942, Carolyn would make her way into the world. This birth was normal and under better conditions than with her first child. Big brother Danny was so enchanted by this little girl that he spent hours just sitting by her crib watching her.

Velva divorced her husband when Carolyn was still a toddler. Velva was left to make her own way, which she embraced. She earned good money as a welder at the Convair aircraft factory, along with many other "Rosie the Riveters" of the day. She loved talking about working in the aircraft plant. She was young, beautiful and independent. She was making it in a previously man's world. Velva was an important part of the American war effort – of American history.

"Convair's buildings were covered with camouflage netting so the Japanese would not see the plant," she recalled. "There were constant reports of incursions by enemy aircraft and submarines off the San Diego shore."

Velva had many recollections of that time – black-out curtains, gas and food rationing, the lack of such staples as butter and the lack of luxuries such as silk stockings. She remembered the fears her co-workers had because they would not have contact with their husbands for months, and did not know if they were dead or alive. She was grateful she did not have that worry.

Cecil Charles (Chuck) Jones was a sailor during this time in unknown Pacific waters. He would write letters home to his parents in Iowa, making it clear that he could not say what ship he was on or where he was. It turned out he was aboard the aircraft carrier affectionately called by her men "The Lady Lex", or CV2 Lexington. In May 1942, he survived the sinking of his beloved ship, but many or his fellow sailors did not.

"We was hit by a Jap kamikaze plane, ya see," Chuck often recounted. "The men down below, those poor sons-a-bitches didn't stand a chance. There was nothing we could do for those poor bastards. We was crippled and ordered to abandon ship so our pilots could finish off the job. We did not want the Lex to fall into the God-damned Japs' hands.

"We lined up on deck, where we ate ice cream. Then, we lined our shoes up on the deck, before jumping overboard. There was other ships in the group that picked us up. We stood on the decks of those ships and watched with tears in our eyes as our own planes bombed the Lex and our home sank into the sea. Ya see, for many of us this was our first ship. For some, coming out of the Great Depression, this was the only home they ever had."

A bond was formed among those men. Theirs was a bond that would hold them together over the ensuing decades.

Chuck an Iowa farm boy who learned welding from the local blacksmith, served on a couple other ships following the Lexington sinking including a repair ship that kept the fleet afloat. They also repaired Merchant Marine ships at times. It was one of those times when Chuck, classified as a shipfitter, was set ashore on a South Pacific island to do welding repairs. The timing could not be worse – a U.S. invasion for control of this small but strategically important island was imminent.

"That God damned Merchant Marine captain put me ashore and left me there. Why, I have never had any respect for those God damned, sons-a-bitchen so-called sailors since. I sought some place to get out of the shelling. Our Marines landed, and I got ahold a colonel who was shocked to see a sailor walking around by hisself.

"'What in the God damned Hell am I supposed to do with this sailor?' that old colonel growled. But them Marines, those boys, kept me safe until they could get me off the island. I am forever indebted to those boys. They have my respect and gratitude."

By 1946, Chuck, was a chief petty officer awaiting discharge from the Navy in San Diego.

Many men were discharged from service after the war, and jobs were becoming scarce for Velva and other women of that era. Convair laid off Velva and the others, and gave their jobs to the returning warriors.

Velva scrounged jobs wherever she could to support her family. Her ex provided no financial support, having dropped out of the picture completely. She worked as a waitress at a popular downtown soda fountain where she learned to make great malts and ice cream sodas. She was a clerk at Walker Scott's, a major department store of the time.

"I quit Walker Scott's when they put me in the pricing room and had me marking up prices for items being put on sale," she recalled. "I just could not in good conscience do that. It was just wrong."

She wound up driving a taxicab, a job she enjoyed. She loved driving and loved the independence the job offered. Velva was a woman with a strong sense of right and wrong. A strong love of her family, she stood firmly behind her convictions. So when the taxi company wanted her to work on Christmas, she quit.

"I was not going to be away from my family on Christmas, and I told them so," she proudly recalled.

While Velva always stood up for what she believed, she was by nature a shy woman, who did not smoke or drink. When her cousin Penny visited from Illinois, Penny convinced her to go to a bar. It was the first bar she had ever been to in her life. A sailor named Chuck came up to them and struck up a conversation. He said he knew another joint they could go to where they could dance.

"I did not want to go, but Penny wanted to dance, and she clearly wanted to be with Chuck, so I went along," Velva remembered. "As we walked down the street, Chuck grabbed another sailor and pushed him off onto Penny, making it clear he wanted to be with me. Penny was not happy. I had no interest in being with Chuck and tried to just make small talk, such as how hard it was to get things like butter even though the war was over."

The next day, Velva's two children came running into the house excitedly telling her that there was a sailor walking up the driveway.

"I looked out the window and said 'Oh my gosh, it's that old chief'," she recalled. "Penny had told him where I lived. He showed up, not with flowers or candy, but with butter. I probably wouldn't have opened the door if not for that butter."

"That old chief" aggressively courted Velva, who kept him at arm's length, despite his deep dimples, good looks, infectious laugh and romantic overtures. A few months of this courting, and Velva told him she had to go back home to Illinois for a while – something about a family situation. She thought he would become disinterested at that point. The months passed by, and Chuck was writing daily love letters. Then the letter came that he had "hitched" a ride home to Iowa on leave and was going to hitchhike to Illinois because he just had to see her.

"Darling,

"Just a line Honey to let you know I am starting for Illinois Wed. morning .... I wish I was there with you now. I sure get lonesome for you, Honey. Hope everyone is well Darling. I have to hurry and get this in the morning mail. Be seeing you soon, Sweetheart.

Love, Chuck"

Velva was in a panic. She was not entirely open with Chuck about the "family situation". Before she met Chuck, she was in a relationship with another sailor – one she thought she would marry. When she became pregnant, that sailor revealed he was married and was returning to his family in South Carolina.

Her plan to take care of the "family situation" was already in motion when she met Chuck. She had arranged for the baby to be adopted through the Door of Hope in San Diego. She went to Illinois to take Danny and Carolyn to stay with their grandparents while she returned to San Diego for the birth. This lovesick sailor did not fit into her plan. She had not counted on his perseverance. She had not counted on falling in love with him. And, she definitely had not counted on Chuck hitchhiking from San Diego to Iowa to St. James, Illinois.

There was no way to stop Chuck from his heart's desire.

"I was showing by then, and I could not hide it," Velva said. "Even this did not discourage him. He not only wanted to marry me, but he wanted to raise the unborn child as his own. I said yes to the marriage, but not to him taking on the unborn child. I had made peace with my decision to have the baby adopted, and I did not want him ever to resent the child. Besides, he was already taking on Danny and Carolyn."

A conversation with Chuck decades later quickly ended before it started with: "Some things are best left alone," Chuck said. A sad look crossed his face before he walked away. It was a look of regret and wondering what might have been.

Chuck and Velva returned to San Diego where the baby boy was born in the fall of 1946. The baby was whisked away to his adoptive home.

"I know I did the right thing, but not a day goes by that I don't think about him," Velva recalled in her later years. "I wonder if he is OK. If he is happy."

Velva and Chuck married in November of that year. Chuck adopted Danny and Carolyn after their birth father died. He loved them just as he loved the third child who joined the family in September of 1947 – Judy Ann. Their family was complete.

FEBRUARY 20, 1999

ON THE THIRD DAY

"Hi, Mom, where's Daddy." Again, I am shocked and worried to hear her answer the phone.

"I don't know. I think he's out doing yard work," Mom replies. "Are you coming now?" Her tone turns worried, almost frantic.

"I'm on my way." I assure her.

"Please hurry," are her last words before she hangs up. Do I hear terror?

It's only 40 miles, but it's a mountain road for most of the drive. It will take about an hour. Something doesn't feel right. Mom answered the phone again. At first, she sounded normal, and then I heard the terror in her voice.

Was Dad really doing yard work? Maybe he fell on one of their steep rocky slopes, trying to clear brush. He might be lying there hurt. I won't let myself think beyond injury.

As I come up their drive, I see four newspapers there in the dirt – untouched. Dad brings in the newspaper first thing every morning. He reads the newspaper, without fail, while drinking his morning coffee. He reads every story on every page and grumbles about the state of the world today. That's how it has always been in our home.

I pick up the papers and notice the oldest one was from Thursday.

Something is terribly wrong. I hold onto hope that he is injured in the yard. I check the orchard. I see nothing. I check the lower part of the property where he keeps his "treasures". Nothing. I scan the boulder-strewn slopes as I head toward the house. No Daddy. The car is here, so he didn't go anywhere. The dreading arises from my stomach to my throat. I swallow down the panic. I have to be strong.

"Oh good, you are here," Mom says rather nonchalantly, as if she were about to put dinner on the table.

"Mom, where is Daddy?"

"I don't know. Maybe he went to the bar."

Suddenly, a look of terror mixed with anger takes over her face.

"Oh, Judy can you go to the bar and get him. Please."

I move quickly through the house. She stays in the kitchen. I enter their bedroom and see nothing. There is an odor. I know this odor. It's one I often encountered as a reserve deputy sheriff. The smell of human death is unmistakable.

Yet, I refuse to think …

I go to the other side of the bed. There he is – lying silently, unmoving, between the bed and the wall. An electric blanket turned to high covers him. His face is covered. I want to deny what I know. I want to believe this is just his blanket tossed onto the floor, or he is just sleeping off a bender.

"Yeah, that's it," I rationalize, "He must have gotten drunk and passed out as he tried to get in bed," I tell myself, ignoring the odor.

I surmise that Mom probably covered him with the blanket to keep him warm, even though we are having unseasonably high temperatures. He just passed out from one too many beers, I'm sure.

I pull the blanket back. I could deny the odor. I could not deny my eyes. My beloved Daddy, my rock, my strength, my pal, was dead.

His body was bloated, his skin deteriorating. My mind flashes back to the four newspapers in the driveway and to that Valentine's Day a week ago. Now I know that look in his eyes was a sorrowful goodbye. At some level, he knew that would be our last day together.

Many thoughts cross my mind. Was it a heart attack? Did he slip and bump his head on the nightstand? Was it … no it couldn't have been suicide? No apparent sign of a gunshot wound. I check his guns. They are loaded as always. No bullets missing and obviously have not been fired recently. I check the medicine cabinet. I don't think any drugs are missing. Why would I even think suicide? Of course, he didn't kill himself. He was too devoted to taking care of Mom to leave her willingly.

"Mom! Oh, my God! Mom has been here alone since Thursday," I say to myself.

The terror she must have felt as she faded in and out of reality – alone here for three days with Dad's body, unable to function, not remembering how to call for help. How many times did she pick up the phone to dial 911, only to forget why she was holding the receiver?

She's sitting at the kitchen table waiting for me to bring Daddy home. I go to her and tell her that Daddy is dead. She cries. Five minutes later, she asks me to get Daddy. I tell her again. Again she cries.

I go into autopilot. I call the Sheriff's Department. I call my sister and my children. I call my best friends Jann and Jeri. I'm going to need their moral support. These are calls no one wants to receive – calls no one wants to make. The calls go on as I reach out-of-state family, friends of the family – there are a lot of friends. I call Mom's pastor and the funeral home. I am in a phone calling frenzy.

Uncle Roy, Mom's brother, drops everything and gets on a plane. He'll be here tomorrow. My oldest daughter Kym is making work and flight arrangements so she can come. My sister, Carolyn, and niece Shea are on their way from New Mexico by car. My cousin John and his wife, Jane; my sister-in-law Marie and niece Tina all arrive shortly to help. More family and friends follow. This is when you know who your friends are. Certainly, my parents and I have many.

The responding deputy speaks with Dad's doctor and the coroner's office. Based on his health, they determine he died of natural causes. No further investigation is necessary. His body will be released to the funeral home.

The funeral home people arrive – the body snatchers.

"Your father's body has been there for several days," lead body snatcher tells me. "That, combined with the electric blanket heat, has caused rapid decomposition.

"We know he requested an open casket, but we won't be able to do that now. It will take a while to remove the body because of the decomposition."

I hear the body snatcher, and I talk to him, but I'm not really here. I can't possibly be here. I feel as though I am in a bubble. There is a lot of activity around me, but as if it is happening somewhere else to someone else. I am just a spectator in this tragedy. The body snatcher's voice sounds distant. An ironic thought, a memory, crosses my mind.

"Dad, are you telling me that you really want an open casket?" I asked as he forced me to go over his funeral home agreement and other things I would need to know as the executor of their estate.

"Of course, I do," he growled.

I forgot I was talking to a man from a Midwest family that took pictures of loved ones in their caskets.

"EWWW," I objected. "I don't want to remember seeing you dead. I want to remember you alive. When I die, I don't want anyone to see me dead. I want people to remember me alive."

This set off a rather heated discussion between us.

"What, you mean you don't want to see me one final God damned time to say goodbye when I die?" Dad angrily questioned me.

"It's just that I'd rather keep you in my mind as alive. I don't want to remember you dead," I tried to reason with him.

"Well, ain't that a God-damned fine and dandy thing," he fumed.

He went on mumbling about Goddamned ungrateful kids. Finally, I acquiesced and told him I would make it a point to look at him in his casket if it would make him happy. But if I go first, he doesn't get to look at me.

So here we are, neither of us gets our way. I am forced by circumstances to see my father dead. An open casket and his wish for his family to see him one last time are denied him.

As the body snatchers wheel Dad's body out, they ask if the family would like to say goodbye.

"No," I tell them.

What am I thinking? Why am I denying my family the opportunity to make that choice themselves? It's just that I've seen so much death, and when you see it, it changes you, even when it's not your loved one. I get very protective about subjecting others to the face of death. It's not pretty – especially not after three hot days wrapped in an electric blanket.

"No. They don't need to see him like this," I say, making the decision for everyone else.

I dismiss the body snatchers.

I go into the bedroom. The carpet is soaked where he laid. The body snatchers cleaned it some, but the stain and odor were there. I open the windows and spray room freshener, even though I know all room fresheners do is add a sickening sweet fragrance to the putrid odor.

Bodily fluids soak the bedding, I notice. Dad must have died in bed. But, how did he get to the floor? I wonder if Mom was strong enough to roll him off the bed. It appears that is just what she did. She probably thought he passed out in a drunken stupor.

I remove the bedding and find the mattress is soaked. I need to replace the mattress, like now, not tomorrow. Can I find somewhere on Sunday to make a delivery? Do I even have the money? I open a drawer in dad's dresser. I don't know why. I just felt guided to it. I open it. There, inside, is an envelope filled with $1,000 cash.

There are enough family and friends here now with Mom so I can go to town to see if I can get a bed delivered today. Daughter Samantha goes with me. Mom has been having a hard time getting in and out of bed, so I want to get a recliner bed, you know sort of like a hospital bed. We find one, but the store can't deliver it until tomorrow. That will have to do. One less thing to worry about.

I return home to find the men busy pulling up the carpeting in the bedroom.

"Wow, there are beautiful hardwood floors under that nasty old carpet," I observe.

"Oh yeah, all the floors in the house are like this except the room additions," my cousin John explains. He helped Dad install the carpet many years ago.

I ask the men to pull up all the carpet in the house. I think it will make a healthier environment for Mom than that nasty, dirty 30-year-old carpeting. I also observe that the flooring under the carpet where Dad laid is stained with his body form. It's spooky to walk into the room and see the outline of his body stained into the wood. It is sort of like a crime scene drawing.

A TIPS volunteer shows up as I'm chewing out Kaiser Healthcare for not putting me through to Mom's doctor. She needs something to calm her nerves.

"Look, I expect a doctor to call me back within the next 30 minutes," my tirade continues. "I don't care if it is Sunday. Don't give me excuses. Don't tell me you can't.

"If you people thought my dad was a son of a bitch to deal with, you ain't seen nothin' yet. I'm his daughter. I'm just like him only I'm much younger so you can't wear me down. Now get a fucking doctor on the phone."

They did.

"Hi, I'm Sharon," a kind lady timidly introduces herself as I fume by the phone. "The Sheriff's Department asked me to come out.

"I'm a volunteer with the Trauma Intervention Program here to help you with anything you need during this time of grief. I can provide resources if you need them. But it looks like you have it all pretty well in hand."

I thank her. Take her information and dismiss her. I think she's glad to go.

No time to grieve. No time to deal with well-meaning strangers. I have way too much to do. Mom, the funeral, the relatives, the friends. I've contacted the main friends and family, but there are so many more contacts to make.

Everyone has gone home now. I am alone with Mom. The cycle of her asking for Dad, telling her that he has died, then grieving again continues. I've lost count of how many times I've told her. I'll be glad when Kymmy gets here. She has always had a special way with her Grandma.

I get her bathed and try to get her to sleep in the lower bedroom with me because of the soiled bed and room odor. She refuses. She wants to be in her own bed. She is afraid and wants me to sleep with her. I glance at the body fluid stains on Dad's side of the bed. I cover the soaked mattress with blankets, lie down on them, embrace Mom and hold her until she sleeps. Does she know who I am?

I'M VELVA DUNBAR – PART III

MY BEST FRIEND

Shopping trips with mom. Those are some of my fondest memories, and most hilarious. We were like two teen girls when we hit the malls. By the time I was in high school, I was earning babysitting money for my own clothes. Mom often matched what I spent, so I had a really nice wardrobe. During the first part of my junior year, we lived in Newport Beach because Dad was working on a dam project in the area. The damn dam, he liked to call it. It was on that job site I learned to drive – and to park. Dad set up two huge earthmovers with a small space in between.

"OK, Yogi," park it, he roared from a safe position away from the car. To this day, I can't parallel park without something huge like a Hummer at each end of the space.

I didn't like moving away from my friends, but I did love the fact that we lived a half block off one of the best surfing beaches in California. By then, I was enamored with the '60s SoCal surfing craze. I was in for a shock and a battle when I started school at Newport Harbor High. Girls and only girls – were required to wear uniforms. This was a public school, and I had just purchased a great new fall wardrobe. Both mine and Mom's school clothes budgets were spent. We could hardly afford uniforms. I was incensed.

Dad didn't get what the problem was. "Just go buy the God damned uniforms," was his reaction.

But he knew it was futile to dissuade these two women in his life when they set out to right an injustice – real or not.

Mom was always at the ready to take on a school she felt was unfair to one of her children. Off she marched to the school, demanding that I not be required to wear a uniform. I was given an exemption. This elicited many questions and a certain amount of bullying from my classmates, but I did not care. Right was right.

I was called in front of the Peer Committee every month to explain my resistance to the school uniform rule. In moments of weakness, I wanted to cave and wear the dang uniform. Then, I would recall the rabid support from Mom, and I would stick to my resolve to fight this stupid and unjust rule.

This wasn't the first nor the last time Mom would battle the school system for one of her children. When Danny's second grade teacher told Mom to not let Danny read so much because he was getting too far ahead of his class, Mom raged against her, and Danny continued to read as much as he wanted and whatever he wanted.

When Carolyn's boyfriend was excluded from the prom because he was suspended, Mom raged. She lost that battle and our handsome Marine brother escorted Carolyn in his dress blues.

And, when my school decided mid-year of sixth grade that I should be placed in an honors class, Mom raged. It was not because she didn't think I was smart, it was because that class was more than a year ahead of the classroom I had been in all year. I has so hopelessly behind that I felt like I was drowning from that point on until tenth grade. Mom's battle with the schools continued every year until I was a sophomore. She finally won, and I was allowed to return to normal classes, where I excelled, and for the first time since sixth grade could exhale.

Up until we moved to Newport, Mom worked as a bookkeeper. But in Newport Beach she stayed home in our two-bedroom apartment. She was bored. She needed a shopping buddy. The first time it happened, I was summoned to the office. I was sure I was again being called to task because of the uniforms. But Mom was waiting. I had a feeling of dread that Dad had been hurt on the job. He was almost killed a few years before when an overhead crane broke loose and dropped a load of steel on him. His hands crushed; he never fully recovered. It was only through determination that he was able to return to work.

"You have a dentist appointment," Mom said loudly enough for the office staff to hear. I was baffled. I had just gone to the dentist. When we were safely off school grounds, Mom confided, "I just thought we'd go shopping and to lunch." This would not be the last time I ditched school to go out and about with Mom.

We moved back to El Cajon that school year after some issues at our house with my sister, who still was living there.

After we moved back to El Cajon, Mom went back to work, so no more school-day shopping trips for me. We, however, had plenty of evening shopping trips including the Midnight Madness sales.

My school had different theme days during homecoming week where our usual dress code was relaxed. A popular theme was Shift and Sandal Day. My friend Linda and I decided we would shop for new shifts. A shift was a straight line, loose fitting, short dress popular with the '60s surfing crowd as a bathing suit cover-up. We forgot to tell our moms until the night before. We were in luck. A midnight madness sale was happening at Grossmont Center. Linda's mom would not take us, but my mom was more than happy drive us there. She loved hauling my friends and I to the mall, football games, dances, the beach – wherever teenagers wanted to go, she was willing to take us – giggling, laughing, yelling out the car window at boys.

Our Midnight Madness excursion turned up a big zero in the main department stores. It was October, after all, so beachwear was not "in". Those New York fashion czars had no clue about SoCal trends. As a last ditch effort, Linda and I went into the Woolworth's five and dime – not exactly the epitome of high fashion, surfer or otherwise. To our surprise, we both found really cute shifts. We conspired with Mom to tell everyone we bought them at Marston's, an upscale store. Our shifts were hits with our friends. No one ever knew they were from a five-and-dime. How could they? None of our friends would admit to ever even entering a five and dime.

Most of these mother-daughter shopping trips ended in hysterical laughter. Back then, my dad was one of the first on the block to have a truck with a camper – remember we were The Joneses. Mom and I took the truck and camper to the Mission Valley Shopping Center, which has underground parking. Mom approached the underground parking cautiously.

"Do you think we will fit?" Mom said.

"Sure, there are no signs warning against it," I said, with teenage confidence.

We drove slowly and without problems until ....

Deep inside the parking area, we turned to go to the next aisle. Suddenly, we heard a loud scrape, a gush of water and alarms. We sat there as a waterfall poured over the truck and into the camper. While we fit under the low roof, we did not fit under the sprinkler heads deep inside the underground parking. We were stuck. Unable to drive forward or backward to escape, we just sat there and laughed. Mall management, security, and the fire department did not laugh, though. The next time we went to that center, we took the car. We noticed new huge signs warning of low clearance posted everywhere.

Our shopping trips were filled with joy and laughter only a mother and daughter who were close would understand. It was little things like purposely putting on ridiculous hats or clothing, trying to find the perfect French dip sandwich, picking out perfect fabric for a winter formal dress, discussing the trials and tribulation of a teenage girl or later a young wife and mom. Dad rarely gave advice. Mom was full of advice – good advice.

She could read your heart and knew how to guide this daughter to be a good person.

One piece of advice Mom gave me set the course for my life. I was 16. We were in the car going somewhere – probably shopping. We had many deep conversations in the car. She mentioned one of Dad's friend's family was coming for dinner.

"Oh, man," I whined. "Their little girl annoys me."

Their daughter was about 12 and followed me around like a puppy follows its mom.

"Well, you know she idolizes you," Mom told me.

Astounded, I asked, "Me? Why me? I'm nothing special and I kind of ignore her."

"Well, you just never know when someone is going follow where you lead," Mom advised. "So, you should always live your life in a way that you will not lead anyone in the wrong direction."

FEBRUARY 22, 1999

BUSINESS OF DEATH

It's Monday morning. I call my boss to tell him my father has died, and I need to take time off. He tells me I get three days for funeral leave. I ask him for more time because I was now left to care for my mother who is in late stages of Alzheimer's. I request some of my vacation so I can arrange adult day care. Max is unmoved.

"Well, we need you here, so you need to get this worked out soon," he tells me. "I can't let you take more than this week off."

"The funeral is not until next Tuesday, I can't possibly come back on Monday," I say.

"I expect you back that following Wednesday then," he relents somewhat.

To hear him, you'd think he was going to have to do my work. Or that I was such a critical employee, the newspaper would not possibly print without me. Never mind that there are five other zone editors to divide my work.

Max never liked me much. He'd like to get rid of me, but I have a record as an outstanding editor, loved by my co-editors, my staff and the public. I have won many awards for the publishing company. He has no basis to fire me. I wonder if he is paving the way to use this against me.

Well, I don't have time to worry about his petty issues. I have far more important things to take care of than my job. I'll talk to HR later. Now, I need to assess what must be done before family and friends return. Let's see, groceries, for sure. The refrigerator is nearly bare, and much of it is moldy.

I tried cooking breakfast this morning and discovered that only one stove burner works. I noticed what looks like a burn mark on the wall behind the electric stove. When I pulled the stove out, I found the electric cord was frayed bare and had scorched the wall. Guess that's the next big item to purchase.

The dryer doesn't work, and the washer leaves a lot to be desired. Since, my condo is sold now, I'll have Guido and John bring my washer and dryer over.

I have to go to the funeral parlor to make service arrangements. Dad and Mom long ago took care of the services. I just have to schedule a day and select a headstone. I will get one engraved with their photo. I already contacted the family attorney. Dad was always hounding me about contacting the attorney the first thing after he died. I guess I have to sign some papers to activate the trust and power of attorney. The lawyer says I don't have to do that immediately unless I need money from their bank accounts. I don't, so I'll deal with that after the funeral.

I'll need to get this house cleaned up, too. Dad would be mortified to have people see the house as dirty as it is. He long ago stopped inviting people inside. It was just too much for him to clean.

The YANA folks called. They anguished about Dad's death. They said they came by the house that Thursday, the Thursday he died. At first, no one answered the door, and they were going to call for a deputy. Then, Mom came to the door. They said they were surprised because she had never answered the door before. She told them Dad was asleep, so they left. Now they are blaming themselves for her being alone for three days while my deceased dad laid there next to the bed. I tried to ease their guilty feelings. They had no way of knowing.

There is so much to do. I cannot spend so much time on the phone. As the news travels, more people call. It's never ending. Too much to do. I hate the phone right now.

WEEK OF FEBRUARY 21, 1999

THE HAUNTING

The house is full of friends and relatives. Some took motel rooms in town; others are bunking here. It's a relief to have help with Mom. It's stressful to deal with the needs of all these people.

Cousin Allen is sleeping in the downstairs bedroom. Kym and grandson Christopher are on the TV room couch bed. Uncle Roy is at a motel. Sally, my brother's widow, is staying in town with a friend. I'm still sleeping with Mom. Carolyn and Shea are sleeping on the family room couch bed. Son Guido and daughter Samantha are at their respective homes. I have no idea where son Jon is. Everyone in place. Everyone asleep. I can relax a little, maybe.

The funeral is tomorrow.

As if the house weren't full enough, someone else seems to be hanging out here. Some believe in ghosts and some do not. As for me, I believe. And, I believe Dad has decided to hang around awhile. I haven't said anything, so as not to spook anyone – pun intended – but then Allen brings up the door.

The house has a front door that is just above the bedroom where he is sleeping. That door is rarely used, and Dad hated it if anyone came to that door. There have been many people coming and going these past few days, and many are using that door.

The thing about the door that has Allen spooked is that he has heard it open and close at night, only to go up and find the deadbolt and chain lock in place. No one around. I have not heard the opening and closing, but I keep finding the door standing open when I know I had secured it.

Then there is the tickling. I woke in the middle of the night last night to the feeling of someone tickling me. I looked over at Mom. She was sound asleep facing the opposite direction. Besides, it was not a Mom kind of tickling. It was the kind of tickle given by fingers calloused from years of work. The kind of tickle Dad used to give. I must have been dreaming.

"Mom, you are going to think this is weird," Kym tells me. "But last night Christopher woke me up laughing. He said someone with rough hands was tickling him. The really weird thing is that I had felt tickling, too, but thought it was a dream."

Carolyn overhears us and says she felt the same tickling. It is good to know dead people keep their sense of humor.

I have a feeling that I have not heard (felt, seen) the last of Dad.

FEBRUARY 30, 1999

RESTING, AT LAST

We laid Dad to rest today. I did not plan any formal reception because already Mom has a difficult time dealing with all the activity and people in the house. Too much stimulation. I don't think she can deal with anything more. She continues to ask where Dad is about every hour or so. It is so difficult. I am not sure she realizes we are burying him today.

My sister Carolyn showed up last night at the memorial, bringing my estranged son, Johnny, along. Johnny is recently out of prison and has yet to repair his relationship with his family – except for Carolyn. Is she playing the one-up game with me? I think she resents that I took her daughter in to live with me when the teen was in need.

I was actually glad Carolyn located Johnny and brought him to say goodbye to his grandfather, who loved him so dearly. I asked Johnny to do the honor of being a pallbearer for Grandpa. Carolyn's one-upmanship – if that is what it is -- failed. I got the last neaner, neaner. I guess sibling rivalry never ends.

A limo pickd us up for the trip to the Baptist church in town. Mom was confused. She had no idea why we all dressed up and were heading out in a limo.

I got up this morning wondering what would be appropriate to wear. I had already moved my clothes to the house. As I looked at my choices, I saw my Class A uniform. My dress sheriff's uniform. Dad was always so proud of my service as a reserve deputy, wearing the uniform seemed appropriate.

Draped over this World War II Navy veteran's casket was the American flag. It made me smile. Back during the Nixon years and the Vietnam debacle, Dad became so ashamed of his country that he stopped flying the flag, something that was a daily ritual for as long as I can remember. Dad ranted and raved about how he did not want a flag on his coffin when he died. I argued with him about it.

"Dad, you earned the right to have the flag. It is an honor. Don't let a fool like Nixon take that away from you."

We had that argument often in his last years. He always won the argument – until now. I made sure he got his flag. He deserves the flag. I hope he was watching. I hope he is not mad.

The pastor spoke fond words of Dad. Some family members worried that he was doomed because he was not a churchgoer.

"Cecil may not have sat inside the walls of this church often, but he was surely a Christian in every sense of the word," the pastor said. "If anything needed doing at the church, needed fixing, he would be there. If someone needed a hand or an ear to listen, he was there. He and I had many discussions about Christianity during these times. I can tell you he was a believer and as much a Christian as I ever met."

I know that. Dad hated going to church services. He felt no need for organized religion. But, he believed. He often talked to me about religion when we would be on family outdoor outings.

"This is where you will feel God's presence," he told me many times. "Out here. Not inside church walls."

My cousin John gave the eulogy. Then it was my turn. I got up and talked a little about Dad and some of my memories. I managed to hold back my tears – my sorrow. As I passed his casket, I paused and saluted. I looked at Mom sitting there, detached -- lost somewhere in her Alzheimer's world. Was the owl calling her? Who? Who?

At the cemetery, the American Legion had an honor guard at the graveside.

It is heartwarming to know how many lives Dad touched. Growing up, my friends all feared him because he was so gruff and swore all the time. He was a hard-working, hard-drinking, hard-swearing man. I see now, most people saw through it all to find his heart of gold. One woman, last week, stopped me in the post office and gave her condolences. She went on to tell me about how he always took time to talk to her and listen to her problems.

"He was like a dad to me," she said.

I heard this many times since his death.

Leaving the cemetery, I turned to see my son Guido, kneeling by the casket. His hand rested on top. It broke my heart. His Grandpa had been the only male constant he had in his life. When I told him Grandpa was dead, I lamented that I did not know what I would do without my rock.

"Mom, I'll be your rock now," Guido assured me. I knew I would need that rock many times in the years to come.

FEBRUARY 30, 1999

UNLEASHED FURY

Family members and close friends gathered at the house informally after the burial. I was hoping everyone would just go on home. I am drained. I did prepare for this possibility and had some snack foods available. My niece, my oldest son and my sister are in and out of the house. They are up to something. I'm not sure what, but no good can come of it, I know.

Oh, oh, here comes my niece and she has her I'm-spoiling-for-a-fight look. She is in my face chewing me out, demanding details about the estate and plans to care for Mom. I am tired and don't want to get into a fight. This is not the time and place for those discussions. I haven't even answered these questions myself, yet.

"I want to know what gives you the right to make decisions about Grandma and the estate. Why are you cutting my mom out?" She is screaming at me.

"I'm not cutting your mom out of anything," I reply, tired of it all. "This is not the time and place for this." I had no idea what she thought I was withholding from her mom. The funeral? That was all planned by Mom and Dad years ago. That is all that had been done at this point.

Friends and family, hearing the commotion, are starting to gather around.

"As for what gives me the right, Grandma and Grandpa gave me that right years ago when they made me the executor of the estate and the conservator for them if they could not take care of themselves.

"This was long before Grandma had Alzheimer's. This was explained to your mom when Grandma and Grandpa created the trust. Nothing has changed. Go talk to your mom. She knows it's true."

My niece looks like she wants to punch me.

"Go ahead girl, you tried it before and I took you down. I'll do it again," I'm thinking, recalling an incident when I was called to her high school because she was in trouble. She tried to punch me as we walked out of the school.

I won't need to take her down. There is a team behind me, led by daughter Kym.

"You leave my mom alone, she's been through enough," Kym fumes as she storms into the kitchen.

"You going to stop me?" my niece challenges.

Kym heads toward her cousin. I have never seen her so mad as she is now.

"I may be little, but I can still kick your ass," Kym yells.

Someone reaches out and grabs Kym before she reaches her target. Grandpa would have been proud of his little Peanuts. The others close in as they realize what is happening. My niece runs outside and tells her mom.

Kym is on a roll today. She has already chewed out her older brother, Johnny.

"How dare you, Johnny, bring drugs into our Grandpa's home?" she yelled at him earlier in the day. I had been unaware of the possibility of drug use that day, although not surprised.

Kym changes from her short tight skirt into jeans, ready to fight anyone and everyone. Meanwhile, the potential combatants have taken Johnny, and left. I think Kym is disappointed that she does not get to punch out her cousin.

The others who are not staying at the house follow their departure shortly. I am relieved. If my sister and niece only knew what it is to take care of Mom, they would not be so anxious to take over. It seems as if it is not Mom's welfare they are interested in, as much as it is the estate, which is much smaller than they think. I will be sure to sit my sister down and show her exactly what is and is not in the estate. I will dot every "I" and cross every "T" so she can never say she was cheated. In fact, I will give her more than her share.

"Watch out for them," cousin Allen says. "Your Dad knew there would be trouble, but you just stand your ground."

I assure him that I am very aware of the issues, and if they want a battle, they can bring it on. Right now, I have too much to do to take time worrying about anyone but Mom.

Mom and Dad's trust is solid. It even has a clause that anyone who contests, questions or creates any problem in regards to the estate will be disqualified as a beneficiary.

There is no loophole.

MARCH 1999

SILENT AFTERMATH

Dad is buried. Everyone has gone home.

It is quiet now. A relief; yet a disconcerting loneliness.

My boss keeps calling, telling me I have to come back to work, or he will have to replace me.

I call HR and tell the director my situation.

"He keeps telling me that I have to come back now, or he will have to replace me," I tell her. "But I can't do that. I have to make care arrangements for my mom, and I have legal issues to deal with regarding their estate. I need more time."

"Didn't Max tell you about family emergency leave?" she asks.

She explains that the federal employment law requires employers to allow an employee up to 12 weeks of unpaid emergency family leave. The employer cannot fire or demote an employee for taking that time. She tells me I have six weeks of vacation and sick pay on the books so I could take the vacation time and add on 12 more weeks. I say I would like to take the six weeks. That should give me time to find adult day care and take care of estate business.

She said she would speak to my boss to ensure he understands the law. I should receive no more calls and need not worry about losing my job any longer. I'm sure this isn't the last shovel full of dirt my boss has in store for me.

APRIL 1999

CONTROLLING CHAOS

I have spent the past six weeks putting my life in a holding pattern. During this time, escrow closed on my condominium, and I prepared to move into Mom and Dad's house in Alpine so I can take care of Mom in surroundings familiar to her.

Caring for Mom and getting ready to put my belongings in storage has been a strain, but there was a lot of help given by friends and family. I don't know what I would have done without family and friends who have adult-sat Mom so I could take care of business, pack and have some brief respite from time to time.

Samantha and her friend Kristen took care of packing almost everything in the condo. That was a big relief. I worry about Samantha. She doesn't want to move to Alpine. It is just too far for her to get to work and school. She moved in with some people from her church for a while. I thought it an odd arrangement from the start. They were odd people. They offered for her to move in rent-free. A week later, they told her she had to move out. The story from Samantha was that a relative was coming to visit. I think there was more, but Samantha has been very closed-mouth. These people are very strange.

Samantha becomes more and more withdrawn. This has to be very hard for her. One day, she is a 19-year-old living at home and going to college. The next day, she is living alone in a condo, knowing she will have to move out soon. She lost her mom, her grandpa, her home and her stability in one short moment. Samantha moved to Alpine for a few weeks after the one-week residency with the weird church people but eventually moved in with her friend Sarah and her new husband. That can't last too long.

I checked my options for adult day care so I could return to work. I struck a deal with the boss to work 30 hours a week, albeit at half the pay. I am supposed to be a zone editor assistant, but I soon discovered I am doing the same work I did as a zone editor, have the same responsibility, all with less pay than before.

Even one of the company executives told me I should file a lawsuit over the boss' actions. I have too much on my plate to worry about his nonsense. I have no time for lawsuits, even less time for the boss. The day will come when he will reap what he is sowing.

Through research and references, I found an adult-day care about half way between Guido's house and the newspaper. So, one of us can get to her quickly if needed. It's priced reasonably and tailored to Alzheimer's clients. I explained to Mom that I have to go back to work, and I was going to take her to a senior center where she would have activities while I worked. If I refer to it as a day-care, I know she would never go.

"Oh, I can just stay home," she said. "I don't need to go anywhere."

Getting her ready in the mornings is as bad as getting kids off to school. She doesn't seem to be enjoying the day-care experience.

"You know, there are a lot of people there who just aren't very smart," she told me one day on the way home from the center.

"Well, you're very smart, so you can help them learn," I told her, hoping maybe that would make her feel useful.

After four weeks of the day care, she is rebelling. She cries when I leave her. The staff says she refuses to participate in any activities. She has become withdrawn.

"She just sits by the window all day and watches for you to come," a staff member tells me. My heart breaks as I picture her sitting all day at the window – waiting. It is the same kind of pain I felt when I dropped my toddlers off for daycare years ago. It is obvious the daycare arrangement is not working. Neither is this "zone editor assistant" job. I resent doing the same work for less money than a zone editor.

I am even more resentful learning that another editor – a male editor – in the same period was allowed to take a flexible schedule to go to school without taking any cut in pay. Makes you wonder doesn't it?

I have been looking for in-home day care. No one wants to come all the way out to Alpine, and no one wants to be there for 10 to 14 hours a day, which is what I would need to go back to work full-time in my old position.

I figured up the cost of having a full-time caregiver while I was at work. It was far more than I was now making at the newspaper. I call Carolyn and propose that I pay myself from the estate what it would cost to hire a caregiver for 40 hours a week. She agrees that would be better than having a stranger in the house.

While I do not need Carolyn's OK, I feel it is important to include her in major decisions regarding Mom and the estate. Despite Shea's suspicions that I am "cutting out" her mother, I am not.

I also include Mom in the decisions as much as she can understand. Dad always gave her the respect to be part of the decisions, even if she may not fully comprehend. He felt it was important to her mental health, to her grasp on reality. I think his doing that helped keep Alzheimer's at bay for a longer time.

It is a relief to have made the decision to become Mom's full-time caregiver. It is an even bigger relief to tell the boss to take his job and, well, and shove it. The day I leave the newspaper business, I will have no regrets. I will walk out of the newsroom; head held high and never look back.

Now the important work begins – taking care of Mom.

JULY 4, 1999

FORCED ISOLATION

Holidays and special events are when I am most lonely. Everyone is out exploring and enjoying his or her favorite activities. It never seems to occur to them to ask me to join in.

I am sure it is not an intentional slight. They probably think, "Oh, well she couldn't take her mom out" or "She wouldn't be able to find care for her mom so she could go."

There are times that is true. However, there are also times when it is possible to take Mom or to find respite care. I take Mom out often. We have gone to the San Diego Zoo, Wild Animal Park, Sea World, the beach, lunch, dinner, shopping malls and to the ranch where I keep my horse.

Neither I nor Mom is imprisoned in this house, as people seem to imagine.

It's not always easy to get her up and going. For some reason, she hates taking baths. And there are times when an outing must be called off at the last minute or cut short. It just needs flexibility.

How many of my friends and family went to the fair, concerts, picnics, fireworks and festivals over this Fourth of July holiday? How many asked us to join them? Just being asked makes all the difference in the world. It makes us feel wanted, loved, alive and human.

Sometimes I feel so cut-off that I feel like I died the day Dad died.

I know I am just feeling sorry for myself. I have many good friends like Jeri, who visit or call frequently. Even some of my Sheriff buddies drop by. My reserve lieutenant, Bill, came by and brought the money collected at the station. I didn't need the money but welcomed the visitor.

I have also lost friends through this. A former boyfriend, Michael, recently went through some difficult times, during which I had his back. When in a computer message I told him about the many friends who stood by me, he replied, "I hope you count me as one of those friends."

"Let's just say an acquaintance," was my cold reply. I was feeling betrayed that I was there for him, but this had been the first contact he had with me since Dad's death.

Others were there for me. Others like another former boyfriend, Carl, who called frequently and sent back a cherished engraved bracelet that I returned to him on our breakup. I wear that bracelet frequently. It is engraved with the pet name my dad gave me – Yogi. I treasure it, and Carl's continued friendship despite the long distance that separates us -- the distance that caused our breakup.

Today, however, I find myself standing at the master bedroom window, looking down the long private road to the house, hoping to see a familiar car heading our way. How many times did Dad stand at this same window, hoping for the same thing?

So, this is what lonely feels like.

JULY 6, 1999

SPLIT PERSONALITY

That mean, cruel "woman in charge of this place" has shown up again.
The "woman in charge" would not let anyone get out of bed, and made them take all their clothes off and run around naked before giving them clothes they did not want to wear.

I had trouble sleeping last night. Mom got up at 5 a.m. again. She was just shuffling all over the house buck-naked. This, after not being able to get her to bed until midnight. What happened to the modest, shy woman who raised me?

I got up and crankily said, "It's still really early. How about going back to bed?"

She did. We both went back to sleep.

Now, as I check on her, I see she is lying perfectly still in the same position, I left her in earlier. She is so still that I bend over her to make sure she is still breathing. She cautiously opens her eyes.

"Is she gone?" she whispers.

"Who?" is my short puzzled response.

"That nasty woman in charge of here who wouldn't let us get out of bed," Mom whispered.

I tell her no one is here but us, so she can get out of bed now. She wanders around her room naked for considerable time.

I had better put some clothes out for her because she seems to be having a hard time with that task today. Some days she can select her own clothes and get dressed. Some days I must lay them out, and she will get dressed. Other days she can do neither.

I leave the room so she can get dressed. Here she comes now, dressed in the clothes I put out for her. But why is she carrying a bra?

"Is this a good bra to wear? she asks me.

"Sure," I say, "but you have one on already."

"Oh, this one? It's the one SHE made us put on. SHE doesn't like our own clothes."

I have no idea who "us" is. I think I have an idea who "SHE" is. SHE is ME!

I tell her that whatever she wants to wear is OK with me. Then she says, "I don't know why they don't put you in charge here, instead of THAT woman."

The battle with THAT woman continues through the day, as I (THAT woman) tire of her insistence that Dad, deceased now for several months, is alive and well, and hanging out at the local bar.

She insists I take her to the bar to get him. I explain for the 999 millionth time that he is dead. Sometimes that brings her back to reality. It doesn't work this time.

She insists she's going to the garage to see if the car is there. She returns and has apparently rummaged through my truck.

"There's nothing out there but someone's truck," she tells me.

"It's my truck, Mom," I respond.

"Well, do you have some kind of papers to prove it is yours?" she accusingly grills.

"Yes, Mom, I do," I say growing weary of this game.

"Well, you'd better get them out," she demands.

I ask her why (will I ever learn to let it go when she is acting like this?)

"Well, you just never know what might happen."

"What? What, Mom, might happen? Tell me." I cry in frustration.

She keeps picking away at this topic, just like she always did with Daddy about finances, about his drinking, about, well, about anything and everything. She can pick a person into insanity. In frustration, I walk out. I go to my computer and start writing. Ohhhhh, myyyyyy, here she comes shuffling in for another fight, I bet.

"Boy THAT woman made me mad," she tells me. "Where do you suppose she came from?"

JULY 7, 1999

'THAT WOMAN' HAS A YOUNGER SISTER

Daughter Kym came down from Sacramento to help out. This gave me some respite. Time for myself. When I came home, all was quiet in the house. But as soon as I walked in the door, Mom shuffled out to tattletale on "That Girl" who made her take a bath.

Kym is reeling between anger at being called "That Girl" and being sad that her Grandma did not remember who she is.

Kym is also very scared.

"Mom, I was sitting on the arm of Grandma's chair, snuggling with her, and then I looked into her eyes," Kym tells me. "I was looking into her eyes and was actually seeing her soul.

"Then I got this awful feeling that she is trapped in there feeling really scared, but she could only tell me with her eyes. That is when I realized that she does know what is happening to her. It is very depressing. But it will help me when she pisses me off like during the bath ordeal."

I wonder. Is that why I never look into Mom's eyes? Do I not want to see her lively soul afraid and locked away in a body that cannot even tell me what she needs, how she feels?

Eyes are the windows to our souls, they say. Today, Kym learned that is true.

It has been a very long day of learning for Kym. She took her Grandma to the nearby Indian casino for an outing. Kym and Mom always shared a love for playing slots. But today, Kym took her there for a walk through the beautiful mall.

"Grandma fretted and obsessed about not knowing where we parked that we couldn't stay long," Kym told me tonight.

Welcome to my world.

JULY 9, 1999

BETWEEN REALITY AND FANTASY

It's been a rough week for Mom. One of extremes. She has either been completely in la la land or completely lucid. I don't know which is worse.

She's not sleeping much again. Consequently, neither am I. I hope it will pass without having to go to a stronger anti-anxiety medication. The stronger ones seem to affect her motor skills so drastically that she falls a lot.

Between "That Mean Woman," the "new guy in charge here," the "people picnicking on the couch," and that whole "big mess going on in the kitchen," we seem to have had quite a busy social schedule.

That Mean Woman hasn't been around lately, but seems to have been replaced by "the guy in charge here."

I was awakened at 5 a.m. the other morning to a banging coming over the baby monitor that I have linked between my room and Mom's room. I rushed to her room to find out what was happening, thinking she had fallen. She had the monitor in her hand and was hitting it on the nightstand. She had never even noticed it before.

I asked what she was doing.

"That new guy in charge told me if I turn these off (referring to the monitor light and the clock radio light) that everything will be OK."

I was able to convince her that the lights were supposed to be on despite what the "new guy in charge" said.

One morning at about 2, I was awakened to the all-too-familiar sound of her room-to-room shuffle.

Upon checking on her, I found her extremely agitated. She said she wanted to know "just what is going on here, with all that commotion." I said there was no commotion. She was adamant that there were lots of people and "all kinds of stuff" going on out in the kitchen.

So I checked the kitchen for her, and reported back that everyone had left, and things were all back in place. That seemed to satisfy her, and we went back to sleep – until 6 a.m. – when she was up and at it again.

YAWN!

On top of the middle-of-the-night shuffles and early risings, I can't get her to go to bed until about midnight.

She sits and reads the same newspapers over and over, all night. Maybe if she turned the newspaper right side up, she would only have to read it once.

On the other end of the spectrum, there are the lucid moments. Often these moments are precious, giving me my REAL mother back for a few hours here and there. But this week those lucid moments have been very traumatic.

The first was the morning she spent in anger and anxiety because she was sure Dad was down at the American Legion Hall getting drunk. She was so insistent that he was there and that I take her to get him out that I had to try again to remind her he died five months ago. She wasn't buying it, so we went to the cemetery.

It was the first time in six months I saw her truly deeply grieve for my dad. Sure, in the past, there were moments in which she would be sad he is gone and would even cry. This time, however, it was complete and utter devastation for her. She also somehow got it into her head that she had done something really terrible that would make him want to die and leave her.

"Oh, what have I done to make him leave me like this?" she cried in anguish.

It was heartbreaking, and it was all I could do to stifle my own tears. But I have no time for tears.

I'M VELVA DUNBAR – PART IV

POTHOLES ON LOVER'S LANE

Mom and Dad's marriage was not Father Knows Best. It wasn't even an Edith and Archie bunker marriage. Shortly after my birth, Dad left the Navy, ready to return to farm life. The Jones family had several Iowa farms including a nice fertile 160-acre farm homesteaded by my great grandfather, August Critzman, near New Hartford. As three of the Jones boys returned from World War II, there was a farm in the future. Their sister, Mildred, already executed a land grab and took the largest most fertile farm. Uncle Paul was already farming, but not doing well. Uncle Glen, an Army criminal investigator, decided to make the Army his career. He was murdered a few months later on a dark street of San Antonio, Texas.

Dad decided to settle his young family at the New Hartford farm. Gramp Jones set about cleaning and painting the three-bedroom farmhouse for this youngest branch of the Jones family. Mom, a former small-town girl, was by now accustomed to city life, having spent years in Chicago and San Diego. But she agreed to give Iowa farm life a try. The agreement was eight years. Dad was sure she would love it. Mom was determined to hate it. Yet, this was the man she dreamed of her whole life. Handsome, hardworking, strong and with good morals, he made her feel loved and safe.

Imagine her disbelief when she found her new home had no running water, no indoor toilet, no bathtub. Cooking and heating were done with a wood-burning stove. The nearest neighbor was a car ride away. New Hartford itself was a sneeze on the map. At least there was electricity.

Farmers' wives were up before the sun – cooking, cleaning, cooking, canning, cooking, sewing, cooking, laundry, cooking, gardening, cooking, ironing, cooking, taking care of the chickens and chasing down three energetic kids and, of course, more cooking. This was not the life Velva imagined when she blew off cooking, sewing and canning lessons by her mother's side to hunt and fish with her dad. She hated cooking. She loved children, but didn't plan to have any.

This was not the life she envisioned as a young woman living in Chicago, dreaming of a college education and a teaching career.

Dad did his best to make Mom happy. Being a man with many skills, we soon had running water and a bathroom, complete with a tub. Not long after, Mom got an electric stove and a furnace. They both worked long, hard hours. My brother Danny had to give up hopes of afterschool activities such as playing his trumpet in the band. Much to the disappointment of the basketball coach, who coveted this new six-footer, Danny was not allowed to join the team. He had to work on the farm.

Mom settled into the role of a farmer's wife, learning all the homemaking skills, including making her daughters' dresses from feed sacks. No joke, we actually wore feed sacks. The sacks were pretty cotton prints and mom actually made us some really nice dresses. She joined and soon became president of the New Hartford American Legion Women's Auxiliary. The American Legion was the social heart of the community.

Velva liked to go to town to buy the feed, and sometimes she was able to go to Waterloo to shop in large department stores. Women were relegated to wearing dresses, even when cleaning at home. Mom apparently like to be cool when she cleaned. Her toddler daughter – me –

often hung onto her dress tail. On a trip to town, while clinging to her dress, I looked up and saw she forgot her undies.

A few days later, the local pastor visited. With childish innocence, I announced Mom's indiscretion to the pastor. Needless to say she was mortified, and I was sent into the exile of my room. At least, I did not get a flyswatting. Mom used a flyswatter to discipline. It did not take long for me to realize if I hid the flyswatter, I would not get swatted, at least not until she bought a new one.

Dad worked long, hard hours on the farm. On his weekend, as much as a farmer can really have a weekend, he was known for hopping on the tractor and heading to town. More than a few times, he drove off into a muddy ditch on the way home after having a few beers under his belt. These beer binges worried Mom. The last thing she wanted was to have another abusive drunken husband. Soon the family had a phone and TV. In fact, we had the first TV in the New Hartford area. The neighbors would gather every Saturday night at our house to watch wrestling, The Hit Parade, The Honeymooners and to play some penny-ante poker. As others in New Hartford bought televisions, the Saturday night parties rotated from home to home. Mom now had a social life.

Mom was adjusting to farm life. My brother and sister had to make some adjustments, but they did. As for me, being a baby when we moved there, it was all I knew and I loved it. If I wasn't at my Daddy's side, riding on the tractor, I was with Mom, or I was out exploring. I loved to help her gather eggs. I loved hanging out in the garden while mom planted or harvested. I loved exploring. Mom took my exploring in stride most of the time. I caused her a few panicked moments such as when she caught me eating an earthworm, climbing to the top of our windmill, licking the salt block with our bull and in the pigpen with new baby pigs. She even did not get too upset when I brought in a handful of newborn mice.

"Judy Ann what are you up to now?" I can hear Mom today, as if she were right next to me. There was a popular song on the radio at the time called Little Miss Mischief. She said it was written about me, and she sang it all the time.

Life was good for a while. Then hard times hit. Dad had been hiring out to harvest other farms after our crops were in. The money was good, and he bought a new bigger and better harvester. While we were in town, after buying the equipment and before there was time to insure it, our equipment shed burned down along with most of our farm equipment and the new harvester. To this day, I wonder about this suspicious fire. Was someone in the farming community threatened by Dad's success?

"This broke Dad financially and mentally," my brother once told me. "After that, money was tight and with Mom on his back all the time about farming, he just lost his spark."

Money was tight. Dad worked all day on the farm, then took a graveyard shift at a factory in Waterloo. I have no idea when or if he ever slept. The pressure sent him to the bottle more often, which put a strain on the marriage.

One day, I saw a man take away Mac our Australian shepherd, who was my constant companion. Mom and Dad were packing boxes. I did not know exactly what was happening; I just knew it was not good. When a neighbor brought me a Persian kitten to replace Mac, and told me the kitten would be my friend in our new "city" home, I knew I would never get to grow up on our farm. I watched out the back window of our Buick as we drove away to a new life.

For the next two years, we lived in Glidden, Iowa, where Dad bought a welding shop. Those who think moving to small town USA is the idyllic life, do not know what they are talking about. Sure, if you have family there already, you will fit in, just as we fit into New Hartford society. We knew no one in Glidden. I was still young, so I was OK. But Mom was lonely, even with neighbors. My sister, by now in junior high school, was bullied mercilessly. Farmers stiffed my Dad regularly for equipment repairs, only for their kids to boo him when his ads played at the local theater. These same kids regularly came to Dad's shop with broken bikes and vehicles, which he fixed for no charge.

Dad's drinking increased, as did marital strife. Mom pushed hard to go back to California. She was sure that would be the answer to all their woes. Dad held tight to Iowa.

JULY 12, 1999

PARKING LOT PANIC

After Kym's visit, I needed to pick up some groceries. I should have done so while Kym was still here. It is so hard to shop with Mom. She won't walk, though she has no trouble doing so when she sets out on one of her adventures down her private road in 100-degree plus temperatures.

Some grocery stores have wheelchair carts that have a basket for the food. Those help, but can also be a hindrance as Mom picks at the food, opens up packages or throws things on the floor.

Today, I only needed a few things, and Mom was pretty coherent, so I left her in the truck. I parked in the shade, rolled down the windows and told her I would be right back.

I was in the store for about five minutes when I heard my name over the loudspeaker.

There Mom was looking worried, with a frantic store manager. When I walked up, Mom looked at me like I was a stranger.

"Is this your daughter?" the store manager asked her.

"Well, no, I don't think so," Mom replied.

"Mom, yes, I am Judy, your daughter,"

"Oh, if you say so," she said.

A customer found Mom wandering in the parking lot, crying and lost, looking for her daughter. The customer was able to extract my name from Mom's confused mind and brought her into the store to find me.

This will be the last time I will be able to leave Mom alone for even a second.

JULY 14, 1999

MIDAS TOUCH

Having been a working mom, and the money manager in the home, Mom is used to having money. In fact, it was always a family joke about how she not-so-secretly stashed 10 or 20 dollar bills in every little nook and cranny of her purse.

When I first started taking care of Mom, I noticed that she spent countless hours going through her purse in a frenzy, muttering about her money.

To ease her anxiety, I started sneaking money into her purse – I try to keep $20 or $40 there. It's sort of a reversal of the old childhood thing of sneaking nickels and dimes from her purse for a candy bar (this was back when candy bars were actually a nickel.)

It gives her security and, also, a sense of self-worth, so when we go to lunch or the store, and she actually remembers that there is money that has to change hands, she will be able to reach in her purse and pay.

As we were about to head out the other day, I remembered she had used her money to buy lunch the day before, so I snuck a 20 into her purse. As I was driving down the road, she was rummaging in her purse to see if she had enough money, in case she wanted to buy something at the store.

She pulled out the 20 and said, "I guess this will be enough; I have $100 in here."

"Wow!" I thought, "A magic purse no less, put in $20 and pull out $100." But, of course, it was only a $100 in her mind.

JULY 18, 1999

FEW UPS; LOTS OF DOWNS

It's been a trying week from my standpoint. All week, mom slid between being angry and hateful, to weepy and hateful. But mostly she was just plain hateful.

Her speech and hearing are becoming increasing problems. Even with her hearing aids in, it seems she can't hear. Still, she does hear, even very slight sounds. It seems more that what is said to her is not connecting in her brain, rather than her not hearing.

As far as what she says ... it's like talking to the Mad Hatter. It's not just confusing a few words here and there – she is completely nonsensical so much of the time, now.

She uses real words, but not so they make any sense in the context – or any context. Then, she becomes angry with me because I can't understand what she wants, or because I give up, in frustration, trying to make her understand what I'm saying.

It's very sad, because Mom used to be my best friend. We would talk for hours about anything and everything.

It's becoming increasingly lonely. I had a wonderful break last Saturday night when Samantha decided to come over for the night. I had her pick up junk food; we watched movies on TV and pigged out. Guido came over to Grandma-sit Friday evening while I went on my reserve deputy patrol, my community service that has suffered greatly since Dad died.

Even with those much-needed breaks, I'm feeling extremely isolated and am suffering a great deal of depression this past week. When people called, even phone solicitors, I kept them on the phone long after they were tired of talking. It was just so good to be able to talk with someone – having him or her understand what I'm saying and being able to understand what the other person is saying.

All week, I had trouble sleeping. Then, I had trouble getting out of bed to start the day once I did get to sleep. Nightmares plague my sleep.

In one dream, Dad yells at me to get the bills paid (how did he know?). In another, I dreamt I was mad as Hell at him for committing suicide. Then he came to me and told me that he now knew suicide is not the answer because it only hurt and angered the ones you love, so I should not think about suicide.

What the heck? His death was heart failure. Why am I so fixated on the idea of suicide? Why would I have such a dream?

I remain troubled by that dream and what it meant. Am I so depressed that I am on the verge of such contemplation? Did Dad actually commit suicide and was trying to tell me never to take that way out? I am sure he did not, but it was a thought that crossed my mind at the time. I don't know, but it is troublesome.

I didn't get a thing done all week, either. I just had no energy or motivation. I've fallen into total lethargy. All of this is coming out in some strange impulses. I woke up Saturday morning and decided I was going to get a puppy. Out of the blue.

I was still grieving that my beloved Persian cat, Shotgun, got outside and was carried away by coyotes a couple of weeks ago. I didn't want to risk trying to have another cat out here. This house used to be the place where all the homeless cats showed up for food and love from Dad. But in recent years, the coyotes have taken over, and all the cats are gone.

I don't know why I decided I wanted a puppy, but I did. And I even knew what kind – a golden retriever.

After I got Dude, I realized there were myriad reasons I wanted a puppy. Now, I have a companion, someone to talk to, someone who never becomes angry with me, someone to run down the road with and play ball with. I trained him to bring in the morning paper without chewing it up first. His only demands are food, water and a pat on the head.

The first night I had him, I slept soundly for the first time in months. When I woke up, I was actually refreshed – a feeling I hadn't felt in more than five months since this all started. I hopped out of bed and took Dude out of his crate and eagerly started the day.

Another big, more underlying reason, was an act of rebellion. Mom has never been a dog person herself. And my dad had not let us have a dog since we left the farm when I was 6.

"God damned dogs don't belong in town," he grumbled whenever we asked. "They belong on farms."

Well, their place in Alpine wasn't a farm, but it was two acres surrounded by acres of fields, rocks and chaparral. It was a good dog place.

When I got Dude, Mom was livid. She blamed her resistance on Dad, of course, saying how he was going to be furious if I brought that dog home. Then, when I tried to remind her that he was dead, she became so angry and looked at me with such hate that I seriously feared she was going to punch me. I wasn't in the mood to pamper her, however, and stood my ground.

"I've given up a lot for you these past few months," I told her, in my best martyr style. "I am going to get this dog for ME.

"I did not get or do things I wanted all my life when Dad was alive, because you always claimed that he would be mad," I ranted on. "I am done giving up things because Dad would get mad. He's dead Mom. He can't get mad."

Besides the depression, I'm feeling a lot of resentment. I miss so much being able to drop what I'm doing and to go to a ballgame with a friend, or meet a friend for dinner or shopping. I miss going on patrol for the San Diego County Sheriff's Department. I miss my sheriff's reserve unit buddies. I miss just being able to go out, saddle my horse and ride for miles by myself. I miss planning and going on my annual backpacking trip in the Sierras.

I resent that I can no longer do these things. I'm losing sight of all the things Mom gave up through my childhood for me. I'm ashamed, but I'm unrepentant for my selfish thoughts. And I'm so worn down by Mom's demands and her accusations. She wore my dad into the grave; I sometimes fear she will do the same to me.

I hide often, where I can cry and swear loudly.

It's hard feeling that way about someone you love; someone who was not only your mom, but your mentor and your best friend. But more and more, I look at her, and I don't see Mom. It's just some strange woman that I've somehow become responsible for. What a horrible daughter I have become.

JULY 19, 1999

THAT BOTHERSOME BABY

I had a job interview today, so Samantha came to watch her grandma while I was gone.

After Samantha left, Mom said, "I'm glad she's finally gone."

"Why, did something happen that I should know about," I asked?

"No, it's just that she had that little baby with her," Mom replied. "She had an awful time with it. She had to sit and hold it the whole time, and it was so fussy."

I asked her, what baby? Samantha doesn't have a baby. Will I ever learn not to try to find some sense in Mom's conversations?

"Well, it's not her baby, it's her mom's baby but she had to take care of it," Mom explained. "It was just too much for such a little girl to be lugging that baby around."

Little girl? Samantha is bigger than I am!!! I didn't pursue the conversation. I was too tired for the Twilight Zone today, besides there are all these other people here today it seems. I have no idea who the "other people" are but there are a lot of them, according to Mom.

So many strange things occur nowadays. In yet another dream haunted by Dad, someone was prowling around outside the house. I woke up with a start. I was sure I heard him outside yelling at someone.

"You God-damned son-of-a-bitchin' bastard, get the Hell out of here," I swear I could clearly hear Dad yelling in his loud, gruff voice.

I grabbed my gun, and headed upstairs to check the doors, set the alarm and throw the lights on outside. The house is at the end of a long dirt road on a secluded hilltop. It can be very scary out here.

Mom heard me and wanted to know what all the commotion was.

"Where's Dad? Why is he outside yelling? Who is he yelling at?" she frantically peppered me with questions that sent a chill down my spine.

Could she have heard my dream? Or was it something else ...?

She was so shaken she wanted me to sleep with her. As if the dream weren't bad enough, I was again awakened. This time to noises at the bedroom window. It sounded like someone trying to remove the screen. This time, I loaded the shotgun and pointed it at the window, finger on the trigger and ready to pull when I saw the face appear. It was the face of an incredibly large opossum.

"Are you feeling lucky tonight, opossum?" I think, laughing off the almost deputy-involved shooting.

JULY 20, 1999

OUR LAST TIME TOGETHER

Mom had one of her crisis days today of vacillating between being angry and being worried. One moment she fumed because Dad must be sitting in a bar getting drunk. The next, Dad must have been in an accident on the way home from work.

It was time for another cemetery reality check. It was another astounding day in this alternate reality in which we are living. We arrived at the cemetery, and I led Mom to Dad's gravesite. The headstone had a photo of Dad and Mom together. On one side, was Dad's name, and birth and death dates. On the other side, was Mom's name and birth date, but no death date. Mom looked at it for a few moments, and then turned to me in horror.

"How did this happen? How did we die?" she shakily asked me.

It took a while to explain that she was still very much alive. That will be our last cemetery visit. I think it is too traumatic for both of us.

To calm Mom, I took her for a ride into the mountains that she so loves. It turned out to be a wonderful day. It seemed like nothing had changed from our days of taking mother-daughter drives for no reason other than to spend time together. I had my mom back.

We talked, we laughed, we confided. I took her to tour the Julian Sheriff's Station where I often pulled reserve duty. We stopped and had delicious apple-berry pie. We explored the town of Julian's many shops.

I felt that I had awakened from a long nightmare.

Only I was living a daydream today and would soon be shaken into the nightmarish reality that had become our life. We stopped for dinner before going home. I could see I was losing her. We abruptly stopped eating and had our food packaged to go. My Mom faded way, replaced by an anxious and confused stranger.

As we headed home, Mom kept talking about how we needed to start looking for a place to "pull in for the night." She obviously was going back to the days when she and Dad would spend months on the road, staying in their trailer. I was now Dad to her. When we got to the house, she wouldn't get out of the car.

"I don't think this is a campground," she worriedly said. "This looks like someone's home. You'd better go check if it's OK for us to park here tonight. "

I dutifully got out, walked out of sight a few minutes, and then returned to the car.

 "They told us to park and come on inside. We'll stay here with them tonight," I assured her.

She never did return to reality tonight.

JULY 21, 1999

MORE GRIEF

Today, we went through a similar grieving as yesterday. This time Mom was more intense and aware than she had been of Dad's death in the nearly six months since. It takes a tremendous toll on my spirit to numerous times daily tell her that Daddy is dead.

Some of the literature I read about Alzheimer's says to play along; don't try to explain things to them. The writers obviously never dealt with anyone like Mom. Playing along only increases her anxiety and anger. She becomes agitated to almost an insane level.

Also, I remember that Dad, no matter how out of it Mom was, would always give her the respect and dignity of talking to her as he had always done. He explained everything to her, making her a part of decisions, trying to help her as much as possible to keep a grip on reality.

I think she would be far more out there if he had not done that. So, I continue his legacy as often as possible, no matter how difficult.

Probably the most difficult part of the lucid hours is that Mom had been an extremely independent, capable, head-strong person.

She was used to taking care of the family finances. During the lucid moments, she assumes she still does. Such as the time she was demanding that she was going to take $1,000 out of the ATM. She became very angry when I tried to explain she no longer had access to the ATM.

Or to driving.

Oh man, driving is a big problem. She has not held driver's license in five years, but she, of course, does not recall that. When I tell her she can no longer drive, she becomes so angry and adamant about driving that she often tries to kick me out of the house. That problem lessened some when I gave Carolyn her car. Sort of out of sight out of mind, I guess. But the issue still rears its ugly head too often.

I remember when I tried to get Dad to have her retested for a driver's license after her driving became terrifying. He was afraid of her wrath, so he did nothing. I, however, being a reserve deputy, had easy access to forms that required someone to be retested. I had no choice. She was becoming more and more dangerous to herself and others out on the road. I never told Dad what I had done, but I'm sure he guessed it.

Mom failed the test – seven times. She kept insisting that the tester was unfair. So, Dad kept taking her back. Finally, the DMV told her, and him, that they would not retest her ever again. She was never going to have another license.

Today, she insisted she could drive and had a valid license. I showed her the seven failure notices from the DMV. She yelled at me that I was lying and that she wasn't the person who took those tests. She eventually went off and pouted. One blessing of Alzheimer's is in five minutes she would forget the whole thing.

I'M VELVA DUNBAR – PART V

CAN'T KEEP A GOOD WOMAN DOWN

One of the many battles between Mom and Dad was over dance lessons. After we moved to Glidden, Mom signed my sister and me up for dancing lessons in Carroll, about 30 miles away. I had dreams of being a ballerina – much like any other girl of that era. Mom saw it as a way of helping correct my seriously turned in leg. Dad hated the dancing lessons and did not even attend our recitals. He thought it was a major con and a waste of money. He also hated having us on the road so much.

His greatest fear was realized one winter night. We were on our way home from a dance class. It was snowing, and the highway was icy. Carolyn was in the backseat. I was in the front. This was long before seatbelts and child restraints, and I usually sat on the edge of the seat with my chin on the dashboard, watching the road.

This night, though, I did not feel well and was asleep on the seat. I awoke to the radio blaring, smoke-filled air and my sister on top of me. Mom was crying in pain. We were hit head-on by a speeding car. I looked out and saw someone seemingly asleep in the roadway. Children were pouring out of the other car, crying and heading toward this lifeless body. Soon, there were sirens everywhere. A man pulled my sister and me out of the car and put us in an ambulance. We did not know where Mom was. No one would tell us anything. I was scared. I am sure Carolyn was, too, but as always she tried to be strong for me.

Days later, after separation from our mom, we were told that we would go home, but Mom had to spend more time in the hospital. She was seriously injured. Still no one told us the details we so longed to hear. My grandparents came to take care of us while Dad worked. We could not see Mom. Children were not allowed to visit hospital patients those days. For two long months, we were left in the dark. There were whispers.

"She might never walk again," I picked up one day as I sat hidden behind a doorway to our stairway.

I didn't understand.

When Mom finally came home, both her legs were in casts that extended from her hips to her ankles. She was in a wheelchair. Her legs stuck straight out. She explained it all to us. She was always open and honest with her children. Both her knees were crushed in the accident. She did her best to avoid the crash, and probably saved our lives, but not herself from injury, by hugging the road shoulder. There was a deep ditch, so she did not pull over all the way for fear of rolling the car in the ditch. The driver who caused the accident had a huge family, and his wife was pregnant. She was thrown from the car and died at the scene.

As for Mom, the doctors said she might not walk again. She would not, could not, accept that. Back then, the medical "wisdom" was to immobilize broken legs, arms and knees completely for weeks, even months. They know better now. What this meant for mom, was that once her casts came off, she had to put flexibility back into her knees. Her legs were stiff as boards, sticking straight out. To overcome this, she spent hours every day, one leg at a time laid over the side of the couch with heavy sandbags hanging over her ankles. She tried to hide her pain from us, but the tears in her eyes and grimace on her face, revealed the truth to us.

For weeks, and months, Mom kept those knees moving and despite the doctors' prognosis, she walked again. I remember watching her hop on my bike, proving she could still peddle. Nothing held her back. I learned a lot about suffering in this time. I learned a lot about perseverance. I learned a lot about strength of character. Just a few of the many lessons Mom taught me.

I never did return to dancing. But that was OK, I had my mom and she was as active as ever.

JULY 25, 1999

GROUND HOG DAY HELL

I try to keep my good humor when Mom constantly asks the same thing over and over, within seconds.

I joke about living in the movie Ground Hog Day, only the character in the movie was able to control the repeated day, to some degree altering the day. I have no such control. Mostly, it's harmless repetition, stirring emotions from amusement to irritation to resignation, such as a recent dinner conversation.

"How'd your meeting go?" Mom asked, surprising me that she remembered I went to a meeting.

"Good," I said, ready to tell her all about my day.

"How'd your meeting go?" Mom asked, not even two seconds had passed.

"Good," I said.

"How'd your meeting go?" she asked again and again.

"Good," I continued to reply, resigning myself to the fact that this would be the extent of our conversation that night.

Other times, it's heart-renching, such as telling her that Dad has been dead for nearly six months. Sometimes it tears me up. Sometimes it makes me angry; sometimes it makes Mom angry. Sometimes even that has humorous moments.

"We'd better wait for Daddy before we eat," Mom suggested one evening.

"Mom, Daddy died six months ago," I reminded her.

"Oh, well, then I guess we don't need to wait anymore for him," she responded, adding, matter-of-factly, after careful thought. "I'll just have to go out and get me another man."

JULY 26, 1999

THANK YOU MY FRIEND

My oldest (as in length of friendship not age) and dear friend Jann drove the 100 or so miles to visit this weekend, despite still grieving the recent loss of her own mother.

Jann has seen me through a lot of difficult times when others turned away. There are not words to express adequately how much her friendship means, nor how much this visit meant.

I didn't have care lined up for Mom, so we bought lots of junk food and makings for my special strawberry daiquiris. We ate, drank, watched TV and talked all night Saturday. Sunday we took Mom out to breakfast then for an afternoon trip to the San Diego Wild Animal Park.

It was a much-needed therapeutic weekend for Mom and me. Thank you, Jann.

JULY 27, 1999

PUPPY LOVE

Since Dude came to the ol' homestead to live, it's been a battle of wills. I think I won this one. For the first week, Mom not only talked hateful about and to my new puppy, she kicked him every chance she had. Not in a way to hurt him physically, but it was still confusing to the poor little guy.

Recently, she was being particularly hateful about the puppy, and I had taken all I could. I picked him up and hugged him,

"If you would just let yourself warm up and love something, you might be a lot happier," I said, letting out a lifetime of pent-up resentment.

I grew up feeling like the also-ran in the family. My brother and sister were more beautiful, smarter and more talented than I. It must have been true since she made it a point to let all her friends know that.

Me? I was "a good kid." That was all. Just a "good kid." Do you know how much I hated being "a good kid." I so wanted to rebel, but it just wasn't my nature. I guess I really was "a good kid."

I grew up thinking I was a twin. My birth certificate showed Mom having four children born alive. My older sister's certificate showed only three. My rationale was that I must have been a twin and my twin was given away or died. I honestly believed that Mom resented me because the wrong twin was gone.

The truth is, a year before I was born, Mom, unmarried at the time, gave birth to a son. She was pregnant when she met Dad. She already had arrangements made for that baby to be adopted. So, I wasn't too far from the truth. Maybe she resented me because I was not that son. I have spent years trying to find information about this half-brother, to no avail.

Don't get me wrong. Mom was a warm, loving person to most people before the onslaught of Alzheimer's. She still has those times of warmth and loving, but there are increasing times when she is quite cold and hateful.

Since my blow up, however, she has actually let herself enjoy the puppy a little. I can still tell it's a bit of an irritant to her, but I've seen her sneak a pat on the head to the puppy a time or two.

JULY 29, 1999

A GOOD GIRL

I took Mom to the doctor today for a regular checkup. She was so cute sitting there on the examining table waiting for the doctor.

She was swinging her legs and looking all around in awe at the posters on the wall. She looked like a little girl about 4 years old.

"Last time I was here, I think I got to go into another room afterward to pick out a prize," she told me, barely able to contain her excitement.

"Maybe I should pick out a roast, and then I'd have a roast if someone comes to visit," she reasoned.

When I was little, I got handfuls of lollypops from the doctor. Mom wanted a roast.

After the doctor came in, she just went on and on about how happy she was to see him again. She told him not to have too many girlfriends (he's married), which gave him a good chuckle.

I had to take her to the lab for blood tests, and she told the nurse there about what a nice doctor she has, how good looking he is, and she was so glad to see him. She gushed like a schoolgirl with a crush on the high school football team's star quarterback.

When we left the office, she asked: "I was really good wasn't I?"

I laughed and said: "Yes, you were. You should have at least been given a handful of lollipops for being so good."

She agreed that she deserved the lollipops. Her tumble into childhood, as in this day, could be sweet and amusing. But for a daughter, it is tragic to watch. I am helpless to control this regression.

JULY 31, 1999

YESTERYEAR

Mom spends more and more time in the past. I'm more often than not, her sister, which sister depends on the day.

Today, my son Guido was here to help with some work. We also barbecued. I'm not sure who Mom thought Guido was. She kept calling him Troy and asking about his Aunt Mable. When he left, she told me how he was two grades ahead of her in school.

Sometimes yesteryear never existed at all. One recent day she began telling me about her two daughters who live in Washington DC, on farms.

"I will be leaving soon," she said. "They want me to come and live with them."

I would have believed her if I didn't know for a fact, I don't live in Washington DC.

Mom never even visited Washington DC. It certainly has been hundreds of years since anything close to a farm existed in that city. And neither I nor my sister has ever lived there.

I have a feeling we will soon lose her completely to the past. It is a devastating reality.

AUGUST 1, 1999

ALL THOSE MEN

In the year prior to Dad's death, we talked about needed repairs and renovations at the old homestead, which had deteriorated a good bit in the past few years.

Although tight with his money, Dad agreed the work needed to be done, and how it would be nice to spruce things up since Mom's Alzheimer's now had them pretty much tied to the house.

We never got beyond the talking stage while he was alive, but I knew what kinds of things needed doing, so I set about getting them done when I moved in as the caregiver.

I've learned I'm a pretty good electrician, even better plumber, installing new fixtures that actually worked was one of my top priorities – just after having the leaky roof fixed. Of course, this is a 50-year-old house, so even the smallest plumbing or electrical fix turns into a major project and lots of cussing – thanks Dad for teaching me how to cuss!

I'm also a pretty good house painter, but I decided I didn't like to be that messy all the time. Besides, Mom would get into a lot of mischief while I was preoccupied at the top of a ladder – it's like having a 2-year-old again.

So, while I did paint half the inside rooms, I hired someone to do the rest and to paint the outside.

I've always liked doing yard work, which here is more a matter of fire safety than beautification. Taking care of Mom and trying to work in the yard prove to be incompatible, so I hired someone to do that project, too.

Along with all these projects, has been a steady stream of male workers in and out of the house for months now. Some of the activities were quite agitating to Mom, but some repeat workers were around so much she began to think they were just part of the family, or at least suitors for me – or for her -- depending on what stage of her life she was in that day.

One afternoon, I had a sometimes boyfriend over for a barbecue.

When he left, Mom said, "Well, we can add that one to the long list of men who have dinner here."

Then there was Jose. Jose painted, put in new tile flooring and did a lot of yard work. Mom was just sure the only reason Jose kept coming back was for me. She finally let that go when Jose started bringing along his wife and twin boys.

Jose, his family and I eventually all became not just employer/employees, but friends. Jose was in his last year of college, then on his way to becoming a math teacher. He, his wife and their twins worked each summer break to save up money for his next year of college. Since he was no longer considered a suitor, Mom decided he was part of the family.

And, of course, I'll never forget the outside house painter. He was a childhood friend of my oldest son. His family lived across the street from us, and I had known him since he was 10 years old. He DID keep coming back after the house was painted, and Mom was quite right about his intent. What business did that boy have strutting around here shirtless, showing off his muscle? Sheesh.

I had to remind him I was old enough to be his mother. This was something that was occasionally a problem with Jon's friends since I was still a teen when he was born. And I have always looked 10 years younger than my age.

One of the hazards of being a caregiver is that people elevate you to a saintly status and put you on some damned pedestal. I've always felt being on a pedestal is a dangerous place, indeed, because when you fall – and you will fall — you get broken to bits. Although his attention was flattering, I had to shatter the pedestal this young man built for me.

AUGUST 2, 1999

THAT'S NOT FUNNY MOM

It's good to know Mom still has a sense of humor, but sometimes it can shake me. Like the day I came up behind her and inadvertently startled her. She turned and looked me in the eyes and as serious as a heart attack said, "Who are you?"

Immediately, I thought: "Oh my, she's even got to the point to where she thinks I'm a stranger."

She's never done that before, though there had been times when she thought I was a sister, my dad and even the governor. Yes, the governor. At least, those times, I was someone familiar to her. So I was momentarily upset when she asked who I was.

Then, she laughed and pointed to my stubby ponytail and said: "I was just teasing you with your funny hair."

That's another aspect of her, now. She can be brutally blunt, like the day we were clothes shopping and I tried on something.

"You'll need to lose a few pounds before you can wear something like that," she offered up.

AUGUST 4, 1999

FALLING DOWN AND APART

Mom has taken several falls since I've been caring for her. One fall, she cracked a few ribs, followed by four hours in the ER, during which she became extremely agitated.

I had to yell at the medical staff standing around laughing and joking, before anything got done. Mind you, it was not a busy ER at the time. In fact, other than about a dozen staffers, she and I were the only ones there.

It's so very hard to protect Mom from the falls. I can be standing just inches away when she trips or missteps. It happens before you can blink. With the exception of the broken rib fall, these are usually just bruising to her ego (and body), and frustrating to both of us.

I don't know why, but when she falls, and I try to help her up, she lets her body go completely limp. I've tried to explain to her how to help me get her up. When will I ever figure out that she no longer has her normal understanding? Usually, when she falls, she refuses my help. She wiggles around on the floor until she gets to a chair, then pulls herself up.

Most frustrating is that when she gets herself up into a chair, she stands up and trucks off a mile a minute, like nothing ever happened, leaving me to wonder why those now-strong legs were like overcooked noodles just minutes before.

Her last fall, however, was one that brought more tears and frustration to me than anything else so far. Perhaps, it was the early hour of 4 a.m. and the fact that I am not a morning person. I awoke to hear her calling for help. I ran to the bathroom and found her sprawled out on the floor. I have no idea how long she struggled there before she called for help. I tried to help her up. As usual, she just went limp – old noodle legs were back.

I sat on the floor beside her, trying a trick I learned about in one of the many Alzheimer's books I read. I then demonstrated to her how to get up on her own. She wouldn't listen. She wouldn't even watch.

I think I will throw out the stupid Alzheimer's books. Obviously, the authors never took care of someone with Alzheimer's, at least no one like my mother.

Mom continued to flail around on the floor like a fish out of water.

"Well, if I can just get turned around to here," she said pointing to the toilet, "I can get myself up."

There she was, scooting and squirming on the bathroom floor, angrily refusing any help from me. She scooted and squirmed until she was right back in the exact position she was in when she began. I told her I was going to call the fire department or a neighbor for help. She was furious and screamed at me. I was so frustrated and upset that I had to leave the room.

I stood in a closet corner throwing my own temper tantrum -- crying and cursing Dad for leaving me with this mess. For about 15 minutes, I huddled into the corner trying to disappear, just as I did many times as a child when Mom and Dad would have screaming matches. I was no longer a strong woman. I was a trembling, confused and hurting child. I needed my Daddy.

I finally pulled myself together and went back into the bathroom. I found Mom still on the floor. This time, though, she was using her old noggin, sort of. She was shoving toilet paper rolls under her butt.

"If I can just find enough toilet paper rolls, I can raise myself up high enough to where I can stand," she reasoned.

It was actually very clever and might have worked if we had enough toilet paper rolls. At that point, however, more than an hour had passed since I was first awakened by her calls for help. I told her I no longer cared if she got mad; I was calling the fire department.

A crew of handsome young hulking firefighters arrived. One of them walked into the bathroom and held out his hand. She grabbed it and stood right up, then trucked off as if nothing happened.

"Apparently, she just wanted to have some handsome men visit her tonight," I told the firefighters.

They laughed and left us.

AUGUST 5, 1999

YOU CAN'T GO HOME AGAIN

Mom is more and more depressed every day. She sleeps a lot. Every time she sits down she drops off to sleep. A lot is due to her medications. I wish she didn't need so much medication, but without the meds, she becomes so anxious you can't deal with her at all. It's a Catch 22.

One of the saddest things is that she continues wanting to go home. I explain to her that she is home.

"No, this isn't my home," she firmly tells me. "I live in St. James. St. James, Illinois."

St. James is where she was born and raised – the place she ran from as fast as she could when she was a young woman. None of the family lives there now. They haven't for years. Her old family home was abandoned and rotting away when I was a child. I'm sure it does not still stand.

Through the years, during summer visits we have watched as the town itself has practically ceased to exist. There is one old store that every so often someone decides to open. It does not last for long. But for Mom, nowadays, St James, Illinois still exists and is the vibrant, Bible-thumping town of her childhood, with a busy railroad station, school and even a courthouse.

One recent afternoon, Guido was putting up a storage shed for me, and I was trying to be of help, as much as Mom would let me. She was particularly anxious and restless that day. She came out looking for me. I walked her back inside the house. Pretty soon, she'd again be coming down the porch stairs.

Mom was being cantankerous that day, though I don't remember exactly what it was all about. I was getting frustrated, because Guido really needed my help. Mom was forcing me to focus all my attention on her.

On one of her trips down the porch, I asked her where she was going.

"Home," she said.

"You are home," I tried.

"No. This is not my home. My home is in St. James. St. James, Illinois. I need to go home."

My heart broke and I am forever haunted by the image of her sitting on the porch steps with tears in her eyes, pleading:

"Please, take me home. Please I want to go home."

I'M VELVA DUNBAR – PART VI

CALIFORNIA HERE SHE COMES

Having convinced Dad that she gave Iowa a chance and now it was time to take her back to California, our family embarked on a three-month journey. Danny was now in the Marine Corps, so it was just four of us. We hit the Pacific Northwest, then back east and down through Illinois to say goodbye to Mom's family. From Illinois, we were on the road to the East Coast, traveling the coast to the Florida Keys, back up the gulf side through New Orleans, Texas – endless Texas, New Mexico, Arizona and finally California. It was a serpentine route.

We camped most nights and had a precision routine where Mom and Carolyn fixed meals, while Dad and I set up camp, which amounted to an old canvas army tent that smelled like mold.

It was the trip of a lifetime. Mom and Dad were getting along much better. Mom was no longer nagging Dad about leaving Iowa, and Dad had resigned himself to heading west. The plan was to hit other states just in case they found a place and opportunity other than in California – Dad's hope, anyway. California was in a high unemployment cycle and housing shortage, to boot.

I think it was predetermined, though, that California would be where we would put down our roots.

California life started a little rocky, as Dad looked for work while Mom looked for housing. We were staying with Uncle Paul, who had settled his family on the outskirts of San Diego. Unable to find work or housing in San Diego, we ended up in Long Beach. Dad worked in the oil fields, and we lived in a small one-bedroom apartment. Carolyn and I slept on a Murphy bed that pulled down from the living room wall. We had no TV and all our personal items were in storage. It was an adventure in boredom.

But Mom would not let us languish in that boredom. She took us to the beach in warm weather, shopping in bad weather. Anything to keep us busy. We were used to seeing Dad with his raccoon welder eyes and blackened hands, but we were not used to the oily mess that covered him on his return from work. I would figure out when I got older that he had to go down into the wells to do repairs. In the meantime, he kept looking for work in San Diego and Mom kept looking for housing and a business venture.

Before long, Dad snared a job at a San Diego ornamental iron works shop. Mom found us a two-bedroom rental around the corner from the house we lived in before moving to Iowa. Together, they found a business – a full-service laundry. Mom worked the laundry. Carolyn and I went to school. It was there I quickly became close friends with a Black girl. Her home was between our house and school. Every day, I would stop over to play at her house, where her mom served us Kool-aid and cookies. One day, I brought my new friend to our house. This was the first time I realized people perceived a difference between us, though I did not understand it.

Mom was very kind and welcoming to my friend, but as time for Dad to get home drew near, she was anxious for my friend to go home. Mom grew up in an open, unprejudiced family. Dad grew up in a family that held many prejudices – really a prejudice for anything or anyone not Jones. Mom wanted to protect my friend and me. No words were ever spoken about our racial differences, and though I continued to spend many happy hours at my friend's house, I never invited my friend home again.

Weekends were family time – working in the laundry. We were closed on Sundays, but on Saturdays , Mom, Dad, Carolyn and I all worked until late in the evening. It was then that our tradition of Saturday nights out for dinner began.

We eventually moved from the San Diego house. Interstate 805 was in the planning phase, and all the property was bought up by the state to raze the houses and make way for an interchange. We found a nice new home on the east side of the inland valley of El Cajon. At the time, it was a rough-and-tumble cowboy town with a real downtown Main Street.

It was a tough transition for Carolyn, but for Mom and me it was just another phase filled with possibilities for new friendships. Mom continued running the laundry, until an offer was made to buy the business. She went back to school, finishing high school then taking college level accounting classes. Soon she was on the road to a bookkeeping career. Dad sweated away in ironworks shops.

Dad was never the same after we came back to California. He seemed always angry – bitter. He no longer wrestled on the floor in tickle matches with us kids. Our camping trips became rare. His joking ways and roaring laughter were replaced by drunken profanity-laced rants and screaming matches with Mom. Dad was bitter he had to leave the farm and Iowa. He hated that he was in California, which he called a "son-a-bitchin' God - forsaken wasteland." He felt emasculated because Mom was working. He felt she mismanaged the family finances. Mom loved being a working woman. She loved being in control of the finances, though she could be a little bit of a spendthrift. Making matters worse was that she was sneaky about what she spent, about what antics Danny and Carolyn were up to, about most anything. But, Dad would always find out, then the fireworks started.

Dad's drinking worsened, especially after an industrial accident that crushed both his hands. He was unable to work for more than a year, further creating for him a feeling of inadequacy because now Mom was the main breadwinner. It caused mixed feelings. On one hand he hated being a "kept man", on the other he was grateful to have a wife who could and wanted to bring in the bacon. He paced the house constantly, going out one door, in another. Watching him would make you dizzy.

The silver lining in this cloud was that during his rehab, he started doing welding out of the garage. He earned enough money to buy a portable truck-mounted welder. He was his own boss again, and he started drinking less and smiling more. Eventually, he was able to join the Operating Engineers Union as an owner-operator and soon joined a construction company that built freeways and dams. Work took him away from home during the week, and he spent many cold nights working. But he seemed happier. He and Mom were getting along.

It was a temporary truce in the War of the Joneses – a war that was all too familiar to the neighbors. Both combatants were loud and proud. Today, the cops would be called, and one or both would be hauled off to jail. But then, the only calls were made by Carolyn and I to our Uncle Paul, who would come and calm his little brother. There was never any hitting, although once, I heard Mom screaming, don't you dare hit me. Hearing that, I burst into the room and got between the two of them. Dad wasn't poised to hit Mom, and I don't know that he would have, but I wasn't taking any chances.

The fights were always the same – money and living in California. There was no variation. Once, angered over Dad questioning where the money was going, Mom took a new approach.

"Fine, if you think you can do better," she yelled. "Then you do it. I'm done."

And when she said she was done, she meant it. She even refused to buy the weekly groceries. This went on for weeks until one memorable shopping trip. I always went with Dad to help. When we got home, she had a friend at the house. She angrily went through the groceries complaining about what a bad job he had done. She pulled out some meat and went on and on about what a bad selection of meat Dad made. Unfortunately, Dad was not making these choices. I was making the choices, and I had selected the meat. I burst into the kitchen. I had enough. I yelled at her for being ungrateful. I told her she was making up her complaints, because I was making the selections based on what she had taught me. She tried to smooth this over with me. But, the damage was done. Even today, I feel the sting of her bitter words.

Their fights were always followed with Mom loudly proclaiming that she didn't need any man; that she would just leave Dad "if not for the kids." Always it was she was staying for the kids. I used to pray that she would leave. I was tired of being the pawn in this contest. I vowed at a very young age that I would never stay with someone who made me so angry and unhappy. I kept that vow and after three failed marriages have concluded I am destined to be alone – and happy.

The peace was broken, and the pattern of their fights changed when Carolyn turned up pregnant and unmarried. It's commonplace today, but in the early '60s it was close kinship to the scarlet letter. Carolyn wanted to keep the baby. Dad felt the baby would be better off if adopted out. Carolyn to that point in her young adulthood had shown little responsibility. Mom sided with Carolyn, perhaps, recalling the pain of giving up her infant son those years ago. This was the lowest point of Mom and Dad's marriage. Mom was unmoving. Dad, feeling he had no option, decided to move out. They were headed for divorce.

I remember the day Dad left, I shut myself up in my bedroom. I was sitting on the floor. Dad came in, knelt down and took me in his arms. I felt his tears run down my back as he held me. I wanted the fighting to end, but I wanted to go with Dad. It was something I had thought about often when Mom would talk about leaving him. I wanted to be with my Dad. Mom loved me I knew, but never as much as she loved my sister and brother. To Mom, I was the talentless tomboy who was a "good kid" but nothing more. But, in 1961, a child going with her father after a marital split was not an option.

The battling continued until Carolyn went to live with Danny, who by then was out of the Marines and living in Iowa – out of sight, out of mind. Dad visited often, and he and Mom would sit on the front porch cuddling and take walks holding hands. It was cute. Soon Dad moved back in. But, when it was found that the State of Iowa stamped the birth certificates born to unmarried mothers with "Illegitimate", Mom brought Carolyn back home, and the fight was on, again. This time, though, Dad stayed. I think he could not go through the pain again. He loved me, and he loved Mom no matter what their strife. Carolyn lived at home for the first year or so of the baby girl's life, and Shea soon captured her Grandpa's heart.

By then, Dad was mostly working away from home during the week, relieving much of the tension. But it was always pins and needles when he came home. Eventually, Carolyn was on her own and with just Mom, Dad and me, peace reigned in the Jones household.

Oh, there were the daily morning news battles. Both Mom and Dad were news junkies. They split up and read the morning paper during breakfast, and the evening paper during dinner, all the while listening to the news on the TV or radio. Both were well-versed in what was going on in the world. Neither was on the same page. Mom was raised a liberal. Dad was raised a conservative. The arguments were lively and many. And, there was a lot to argue about back then – Vietnam, the draft, Civil Rights, Women's rights.

Ask me where I stand politically – and you will find a middle-of-the-roader, who can argue either side. Although, I suppose I leaned more toward Mom's side. She became active in Democratic politics and often took me along while she campaigned. I started walking the campaign trail with her at 12 during John F. Kennedy's presidential run. Before I was even 21 – then the voting age -- I was a precinct captain for Robert F. Kennedy. Mom didn't just work for major campaigns; she was active with local, state and minor federal campaigns. She even ran for local office and was elected to the San Diego Democratic Central Committee where she served many years as the treasurer. She was a tireless crusader against over-development. She remained active until she and Dad both retired and started RVing around the country.

What tickled me the most about Mom's retirement was when I learned she was going to Garden Club meetings. Garden Club was not exactly the type of activity you thought of when you thought of Mom. In fact, my brother called her the Gray-haired Hippie, when she took up dirt bike riding with my Dad. Nothing could slow Mom down, not the reins of a small-town conservative society, not a bad love affair, not broken knees – nothing, until ... Alzheimer's. The battle she would only win in death.

AUGUST 6, 1999

SCREAMING KID & OTHER NUISANCES

Well that unruly kid came back to torment Mom today.

I'm not sure, but I believe the "screaming kid" she heard this time, was actually the electric screwdriver Jose used to put in backing for the kitchen tile.

She just kept going on and on about that "screaming kid" and how she would paddle its bottom if it were her kid.

Later, in the quiet of the night, she said, "I'm sure glad they finally took home that screaming kid."

We also have had a lot of partiers lately, who insist on having their parties here at the house. This annoys her greatly. What annoys me is that they aren't inviting me to their parties.

Maybe I am not invited because the last partiers, real ones, at a neighbor's house decided to use Mom's driveway as their parking lot. I greeted them with my Glock in hand.

I don't know, but it seemed like Dad took over my body that night as I told them in no uncertain terms to get off our property. I am mostly seen as soft spoken, maybe even gentle in some ways, but when I need it, I can dig deep down into my soul and pull out a command presence that those who have seen it, never forget.

Maybe the word is out not to invite the crazy gun slinging woman at the end of the lane to any parties, not even imaginary parties.

AUGUST 7, 1999

WHAT'S THAT YOU SAY?

I am now completely convinced that Mom's hearing problem is an understanding problem. She can hear just as good without her hearing aids as when she wears them. It just depends on if her brain is making the connection with her ears or not, as to whether she "hears" what you say.

So, since she lost one hearing aid the other night, I've not had her wear the other. She hears (understands) me at the same rate. I am not sure where the hearing aid went. She may have put it anywhere.

A couple of days before she lost it, an electrician friend was over checking out the aging wiring, and Dad's creative fixes, that had me worried. As he walked around the house, we kept hearing a squeal. I checked Mom's ears and discovered one of the hearing aids was missing.

Steve and I set out on a search for it. As we traveled around the house on this mission, the squeal seemed to be following us. Steve turned his back toward me, and I burst out laughing – Mom had dropped her hearing aid into his tool belt.

"I thought she was just trying to pat my butt when she walked by earlier," Steve joked.

Knowing how Mom sometimes thinks she is still a young woman, and how man crazy she was, she may have actually been trying to pat his butt when she lost the hearing aid. Steve does have a nice butt.

AUGUST 8, 1999

STRANGE BREW

Besides strange conversations, Mom is concocting strange drinks. Her interesting, if not tasty, drink recipes started before Dad died. I remember one day we were all at the table, and she took Mrs. Dash seasoning and poured it into her glass of water. Worse yet, she drank the whole thing and commented on how good it was. We took her word for it.

She's always adding peanuts, candy and cookies to whatever she happens to be drinking, so I've gotten used to these strange brews. Tonight, however, was more than I could stomach. I was getting dinner on the table when I noticed her dropping chocolate candies into a mixture of coke, water and tea. I then noticed something white in the bottom. On closer look, I found she had dropped a piece of chicken meat into the mixture.

As funny as her barista recipes are, they can also be scary. I have to be very careful not to leave any cleaners out because I have caught her trying to put household cleaners into her drink. I think, just like a toddler, when she sees the pretty blue and purple colors, she thinks they are soda pops.

I also must watch her closely during meals because she sticks food into her bra. It is not unusual when undressing her at night to find cookies, chicken, sandwiches – whatever we happen to have to eat that day – in her bra.

And I thought when my last baby left home, I didn't have to worry about such things anymore. I can't ever get a break.

PART II

PAINFUL CHOICES

My return to work, a difficult journey for my sister, and a continued degradation of Mom's condition force us to make some difficult decisions—decisions we do not want to face; ones that bring us pain, guilt, tears and ... relief.

AUGUST 9, 1999

MOVIN' ON

I just got back from a job interview with the City of El Cajon Police Department for a non-sworn position as a police service officer. It was my final interview and was with the Chief of Police.

When I applied for this job, I didn't really think I would get hired because these jobs were usually filled internally. But it's looking good.

This would be a great place for jumping off the sinking newspaper ship.

I've lost my love for journalism. Broadcast media has changed newspaper journalism for the worse. Instead of focusing on good, local reporting – the mainstay of newspapers – print media have tried to become like broadcast news – shallow entertaining clips with just enough of a glimpse of real news to call themselves journalists.

I hate the sensational angles. I hate playing loose with the facts, with the truth. I hate downplaying important, real news, while up-playing mindless fluff. I hate the nasty, cutthroat business of journalism of today.

More and more, I identify with my law enforcement side. This will be a good thing if I can get the job with the PD. I'll be close to Mom's house. I'll have better pay and benefits. I will have stable hours. And, I will have less stress.

The chief said I should hear in a week if I am selected. I'm not sure what I'm going to do about Mom's care at this point. I'll worry about that if I get the job.

AUGUST 16, 1999

YOU'RE HIRED!

I hadn't heard from the police department, so I called personnel today. The clerk said: "Oh, didn't anyone call you? You've been hired."

"Really? Uh, when do I start?"

"When do you want to start?"

OK. Sort of odd. I decided to start the job in two weeks to give me time to arrange for Mom's care.

Carolyn said she wants to come to take care of Mom while I go back to work. Since her husband, Jim, is a long-haul trucker, he isn't home that much. She said she can stay here and go back to New Mexico whenever he comes home. It's a relief because I could not find any in-home care people who wanted to come out to Alpine.

There is a big, HOWEVER. My sister doesn't stick to things for long. I've already heard that family friends and family members are taking bets on how long she will stay.

Seems no one thinks she'll go beyond a week. Nevertheless, I'm going to move forward, and plan on her being here for at least a month. Then maybe I can figure out another arrangement.

AUGUST 18, 1999

TRAILER FOR SALE, DATE INCLUDED

I bought a used travel trailer this week. No, I don't plan to hit the road
– although there are times when that sounds like a good idea.

I'll be going back to work full-time soon (none too soon to be truthful).
I need to prepare for my sister's arrival. Carolyn lives about nine hours
away. Mom's house is large, but only has two bedrooms, and besides, as
much as Carolyn and I love each other, we have had fights that turned
physical. The brawling Jones girls.

To avoid that outcome, we decided a used travel trailer would be a
good investment. She told me she'd trust my judgment on buying a
suitable one. I found a trailer, and it came with a bonus. It came with a
suitor. And this suitor seems to be a rather unusual man, indeed.

I've had male friends (one an off-and-on boyfriend) come to the house
to visit or call me regularly since Dad died, turning my life upside down.

The closest I've come to being asked on a date is: "I'd take you to
dinner, but I know it's a problem to find care for your mom."

Even assurances that I could get care, never led to an actual firm offer for a date. I think they just used my mom as an excuse to avoid a date altogether. So, you can imagine my surprise, when the gentleman, whom I purchased the trailer from, called to chat the very next day, and then asked if he could take me and Mom to a champagne brunch on Sunday. Of course, I said yes.

I had no idea if this first date would be the last or if there would be more, but I have to say the man was starting off on the right foot by solving the Mom problem – and on a first date no less. Now that is a gentleman with class.

Phil returned several times to visit. We spent one pleasant evening sitting on top of the largest of the boulders surrounding Mom's patio, sharing a bottle of wine and watching the sunset.

"I love this so much," Phil said, pensively. "But one day, I just might not come back."

"Why is that?" I asked, feeling nervous that this might end before it starts.

"I have my business here, but my home is in Mexico," said this obviously non-Mexican man.

A story then unfolded of parental kidnapping, ties to powerful Mexican government officials, and regret that he cannot stay in the States much longer.

I choke down a lot of emotions. Here I am, a deputy sheriff, who has just been told about a crime. What was I supposed to do with this information? How was I supposed to react?

I was surprised at his candid conversation. He knew I was a deputy. Why did he have to tell me? It was a crime that was ages old. His ex-wife was a drug addict and was abusing their son, who is now an adult in his 30s. Phil took the boy when he was just a toddler and headed south, never to return to live in the States.

I just listened, saying nothing. I'm sure he read my thoughts. The sun was setting on the sunrise of our friendship, as we sat silently together, on that boulder on top of the hill drinking our wine. We both knew this would be our last time together. Our last conversation.

I am forever grateful for the brief respite Phil brought from being alone with Mom. I am sad it was so short, but relieved that Phil did the right thing by not coming back. By not making me choose between him and my duty as a deputy. He may be one of the few remaining good guys in this world, despite his past.

LATE AUGUST 1999

SO FAR, SO GOOD

So far, Carolyn is working out. I think it's good she is here so she can see how difficult it is to watch Mom drift further and further away from reality. There is not much reality left around here.

This time has also allowed for some healing of bad feelings between my sister and me that have festered over the past few years. When we were growing up, I felt lost in her shadow. She was model beautiful and talented at everything she undertook. I was a freckle-faced tomboy with no talent. I guess part of me was always envious of the attention Mom gave her.

Carolyn is five years older than I. While her life fell apart, she guided me. She set me on the right path and ensured I stayed there. For that, I am thankful.

We mostly shared bedrooms as kids, and we used to have a lot of deep conversations when we went to bed. Now, she answered some troubling questions for me about things that happened to her, and may have happened to me. Things so private that I could never talk about them with anyone else.

Somewhere along the line, Carolyn chose a very different path. I won't say the wrong one, just different. As a result, she has ideas and quirks that would seem odd to many. That's the way it is with truly creative people.

Yet, I don't understand why Carolyn won't sleep in a bed. I got the trailer so she can have her own space. I spent hours cleaning it up and replacing curtains and seat covers. It's a nice comfortable trailer. But she isn't interested.

The trailer, which I thought would be a place for Carolyn to get away for some respite, turns out to be a place for me, instead. I hide there when I need a break from the insanity. Carolyn hasn't set foot in it.

She'll sleep on the couch, even though there is an extra bed since lately Mom won't sleep at all if I don't sleep with her. So every night, Carolyn curls up on the couch, and I squeeze into the double bed with Mom. Sometimes Mom turns and just holds on to me. I think she is very afraid. I am not sure what causes her fear. Is it losing grip on who she is? Is it fear of dying? She once told me she was afraid of death. That made me afraid. It seemed cold and empty. A dead end on the soul's journey.

EARLY SEPTEMBER 1999

THE HONEYMOON IS ALMOST OVER

I don't think Carolyn is going to last much longer. Having her here has not been much of a relief for me. Sure, I can go to work knowing Mom is cared for, but I must rush home to take over and relieve Carolyn because Carolyn gets stressed.

Carolyn only stayed over one weekend, so I have no weekend breaks. If I'm late even a few minutes, Carolyn is calling me wanting to know when I will be home. As soon as I walk in the door on Thursdays (I work four days a week) she beats feet out whether her husband is home or not.

The stress is too much. I'm the bomb-proof one. I should have known this would be hard for her. It's hard for me, and I'm not as nervous and high strung as Carolyn. I am not getting any respite at all. Bomb-proof or not, I'm exhausted and lonely.

I am grateful for the time of sisterhood healing we have had. That is the good part about family crises; you are forced together, sometimes an uneasy truce is formed, sometimes wounds are healed, and relationships are restored. At least for the moment.

LATE SEPTEMBER 1999

LOSING CONTROL

Mom is starting to get out of control. Along time ago, I had to secure the house with locks and an alarm system to keep her from wandering off. It worked for a while, but now she throws tantrums when she can't get out.

The other night, after Carolyn left, she was screaming, pounding and kicking doors and windows. Then she started throwing things at the windows, including a kitchen chair. Who knew an 84-year-old woman had that kind of strength?

I reverted to my childhood behavior, cowering in a closet terrified, alone and crying hysterically just as I did when she went into these rages at Dad. I can't live with this kind of terror much longer. I feel myself reverting to childhood more and more.

The other day, as I tried to bring Mom inside the house, she turned on me. She was hitting, swinging at me, trying to land a punch. I cannot fight back or restrain her because I am afraid I will hurt her. She may be strong, but I am stronger. Her aggression is growing daily.

I look into Mom's eyes, and I can no longer find even a flicker of my mom. I think back to bruises and cuts, including a black eye that my dad sported. The explanations were reminiscent of those I would hear as a deputy on domestic violence calls. "Oh, I slipped and fell," "I got clumsy and walked into a door," etc.

I never made the connection between those victims' excuses and the reasons my dad provided for his injuries. Now, sadly and deeply regretful, I know he was being physically abused. My heart breaks at how alone he was. None of us realized it. And, he was too proud to tell us.

Speaking of losing control, Mom has other control issues, now. On the way home from an outing, just minutes from arriving, Mom had a bowel movement that she could not control. My new truck's seat will never be the same.

She was mortified, and squirmed all around, which made matters much worse. By the time we reached the house, she was covered in it. I didn't want to have it tracked into the house, so I stripped her down on the patio and hosed her off. It seems cruel, but I couldn't think of any other way. I bundled her up and rushed her inside where a nice warm bath was the next step.

Then there was the trip to her favorite buffet. She sat down with her plate, took one bite, gagged and threw up all over the table. She has problems with eating sometimes because an uncontrollable gag reflex takes over. Usually, when she is anxious this happens, and, nowadays, she gets anxious whenever we are away from home.

I sought out the manager and found an assistant. I explained what happened and asked if I could prepare a plate to take home so she could try eating again later.

"Oh no, I can't let you do that," he said, obviously repulsed by the situation.

"The sign when you come in explains that you can eat all you want, but you have to eat it here," he added with haughty airs that might be appropriate in a four-star restaurant, but not in a buffet with marginally edible food.

"You can make her as many plates as you want, but she has to eat it here," he firmly stated.

But wait, he just didn't know with whom he was dealing.

"Look, my mom has been coming here with my dad for years, at least once a week," I told him, deliberately loud enough for nearby diners to hear. "He died recently and she is suffering from Alzheimer's. She's mortified at what's happened. Can't you make an exception? And if you can't, then get me a manager who can," I added, my voice now rising and some swear words that would make Dad proud are on the tip of my tongue.

The manager came over to the table, also obviously appalled that Mom had vomited all over his table.

"I'm going to have to ask you to take her out of here," he demanded loudly enough to embarrass Mom.

"Hey, we want to get out of this God damned place as badly as you want us out, but we paid for your fucking overpriced food, and all I'm asking is to take one plate of food home where she won't be so anxious and will be able to eat."

Those words that would make Dad proud flew off the tip of my tongue into the now-silent air as customers stopped their jabber to watch the unfolding drama. The jerk held out, but in his eagerness to remove us without having to call the cops (it wouldn't have helped him much since I know all of them), he gave me gift cards for two meals, and shoved us out the door.

I should have reported him to his corporate office because his behavior was not befitting a joint that purports to be THE family place to eat. But as with other things, nowadays, I have enough to stress about. I just didn't need to take this any further – for my own sake, not his.

LATE SEPTEMBER 1999

THIS HONEYMOON IS REALLY OVER

Carolyn told me she can't do it any longer. She made it longer than most of us thought she would. That abandonment, combined with Mom's escalating aggression and rapid deterioration has caused me to think about the unthinkable – a care facility.

It's such a painful choice. Mom was always terrified that she would end up in a facility the way her mother did. Grandma had dementia also. It was not officially diagnosed as Alzheimer's, but the same symptoms were present.

I remember traveling to Illinois to see Grandma when she was at the "home." She had pulled out all her hair and picked sores on her body. She was bedridden. I don't want to see my mom that way. How can I do that to my own mother?

My heart is breaking. The guilt is unbearable.

Dad used to say, "I know when we can't take care of ourselves, you God damned kids are just going to lock us up in some shit-hole home and forget us."

I would promise him I wouldn't let that happen. Now it seems I was being faced with doing just that.

END SEPTEMBER 1999

THE HUNT IS ON

I checked facilities I was referred to by friends, relatives and doctors. Several people told me about one in Alpine, the Alpine View Lodge, just down the road from Mom's house. Everyone spoke highly of the place.

Carolyn and I took a tour. This was a decision I was not going to make alone. It was a small facility and housed only mobile Alzheimer's residents. Each resident has her own room and shares a bathroom with one other person. They can decorate the room in any manner they wish, even bringing in their own furniture. Some even have small pets such as birds.

They have plenty of activities. You never see people listlessly sitting around. There is a community garden, a beauty shop and a home-style "restaurant". You can visit at any hour, without any kind of advance notice. There are weekly ice cream socials for family members and other activities to include the family. I think Mom will like it – I hope.

There was a man there, also taking a tour. His wife has Alzheimer's. He asked about being able to move there with her. He had tears in his eyes as he walked listlessly through the place. You could feel his pain. I thought of

Dad. How he would have felt if he had lived to see this ending for Mom. Is he in Heaven, hating me for doing this? Or is he relieved that he did not live to make the decision? I will make it a point to tell my kids to just put me away if I get Alzheimer's. I do not want them to feel this guilt. I am giving them permission while still of sound mind.

EARLY OCTOBER 1999

IT IS DONE

The decision has been made. Mom was moved to her new "home." I wasn't strong enough to do this myself. Thankfully, Carolyn and my niece Shea volunteered to move Mom. Carolyn knew it was tearing me up. For all our disagreements and differences, I can usually count on her when I am most desperate – and I am desperate.

I came home from work tonight to a silent house. Mom is gone. Carolyn is gone. It is so lonely. I called Carolyn to ask how it went. She said Mom fought it when she was told she was going to be staying there. She told me that Mom cried and said, "My daughters wouldn't do this to me."

Did Mom really say that? That sounds too rational for her current phase of Alzheimer's – the stage where there are no more lucid moments. But, still, those words haunt me. They will haunt me for a long time. Probably forever.

We were told we shouldn't visit for the first month. They want her to get used to living there. I just want to go hold her and tell her I love her, tell her how sorry I am, and that it is going to be OK. But is it? Will it ever be OK? I want to bring her home.

It's quiet and lonely here at Mom and Dad's home. This is the first I've really had time to grieve for Daddy. I dug out his Navy pea coat and wrapped myself in it. My mind wandered back to my childhood, to this handsome Navy chief who held me firmly in his arms as I found comfort snuggling into the shoulder of this very coat.

I see him walking the floor with me when I was sick and unable to speak. I would open my mouth, but no sound came out. I was terrified but was comforted by his calmness, his strength, his assurances. I can smell and feel all of that wrapped up now in his coat. He is here with me.

NOVEMBER 1, 1999

THE FIRST VISIT

I visited Mom today. The first time, since moving her to the facility. Carolyn is back in New Mexico, so I went alone. I sat in the parking lot for a long time, getting my emotions under control, and my courage up. Would she remember me? How was she going to react? How was I going to respond? It was family ice cream social day. She loves ice cream, as do I. It will be OK.

She was in the main lobby. I stopped at the door and watched her. She sat alone. She looked sad. I came to her, but she never looked at me. She recognized my voice. I think. At least I saw what I hoped was a flicker of recognition.

She shunned me.

She looked great. Carolyn had arranged for her to have weekly hair appointments in the beauty shop, something Mom always did before Alzheimer's.

She followed me to the ice cream social and enjoyed her ice cream, even if she wasn't enjoying me. She never said a word. Never made eye contact. Mom was always good at silent treatments and guilting. She stopped talking to me for two months once because I questioned her use of so many prescription medications. I was getting a full dose of it today. I guess I deserve it. I spent most of the day with her, but she never acknowledged my existence. Maybe next time.

MID-NOVEMBER 1999

WE'RE OUTTA HERE

I continue to visit Mom regularly and always to the same icy treatment. I thought maybe if I broke her out of the place she would accept me again. She is allowed to be taken on outings, even overnighters, but I have been afraid to try it on my own, so I enlisted Samantha's aid. My cousin, Mary, had given me a wheelchair, which Mom would never use when at home. This time I had leverage.

"Do you want to go to the beach?' I asked.

"Oh yes," she said.

"Well, then, you will ride in a wheelchair, or you don't get to go."

That strategy worked to get my kids in strollers when they were little, and it worked on Mom. She complied, grudgingly. We had a lovely day cruising the boardwalk at Mission Beach, about an hour's drive from Alpine. She was reluctant to go back to the home, but didn't give me too much trouble.

The outing was what she needed – what we both needed.

THANKSGIVING 1999

"SUCH A BEAUTIFUL HOME"

The home had holiday meals for all the family and encouraged me to have the family join Mom there. They explained that the holidays are very stressful times for those with Alzheimer's and advised me it would not be a good idea to bring her home. I compromised with them. I would bring her to her house on Thanksgiving, and on Christmas, we would celebrate at the home.

I was planning to keep Mom all night. I made sure that the meal was already prepared before I picked her up, so she wouldn't feel like she needed to do anything but enjoy the food and the family. I was eager for her to see the house. All the renovations were complete, and the house looked great.

After dinner, I found Mom standing by one of the many windows looking out across the valley below.

"You have such a beautiful home," she told me.

"Well, Mom, this is your home. Remember, the home where you and Daddy lived for 30 years?" I reminded her.

"No, no, this isn't my home," she said.

Shortly after, she began to demand I take her home. I said I would. I hoped she didn't think I was taking her to St. James, Illinois. When we got to the care center, she said it wasn't her home. I told her it was. That was that. She accepted it and allowed me to take her inside.

We had several more outings after Thanksgiving. When my daughter Kym came from Sacramento, she, Samantha and I took Mom to the San Diego Zoo. We had a great time, laughing until we cried as we wheeled her around. We were hysterically laughing as we headed down one of the many steep trails, not recommended for wheelchairs. They need to put that warning at both ends of the trail.

We wheeled down at breakneck speed, nearly losing control more than once. Fortunately, there were three of us to keep from losing grip on the wheelchair. Although, in the end, we came to such a quick stop, we almost dumped Mom onto the ground. She gave us that look we used to get when we did something wrong as kids.

It was good to laugh again.

DECEMBER 1999 & BEYOND

FAMILY, FORGIVENESS & SHENANIGANS

For Christmas celebrating, I decided to take the home's recommendation to bring Christmas to Mom, instead of Mom to Christmas. The Thanksgiving celebration at home was stressful for Mom – and the family.

The week before Christmas, the home holds a family celebration. Tree decorating, dinner, and gifts are on order for the families.

Each family had its own table for Christmas dinner, which was served family style. After dinner, we strolled around the grounds. Mom looped her arm through my son Guido's and struted proudly past her envious neighbors.

She was oblivious to the rest of us. I think she was again a beautiful young woman strolling through the park with her handsome beau.

By now, Mom seems to have accepted that she lives at the home. Perhaps, she no longer remembers living anywhere else. I think she has forgiven me for moving her there. Or maybe she just doesn't remember.

At least she talks to me, now. In recent visits, she has filled me in on the "locals" and local gossip. There's a doctor there, and he was once really a successful doctor.

"He's a doctor," she tells me, pointing at the little old man walking by. "He's a widower, too."

"Oh, really? So is he your boyfriends?" I tease.

"Oh, no," she blushes. "He's too handsome. He'd never look at a freckle face like me."

Mom never realized just how beautiful she really was and still is.

It is very interesting watching the dynamics at the home. One afternoon, I saw four of mom's female neighbors standing in a group whispering. Mom said they were the popular girls and thought they were better than everyone else. I moved closer to listen in. I'm not nosey, I just have journalistic inquisitiveness.

"OK, so I know where there is a party tonight," the ringleader, one-time teacher, told her gang. "We will have to wait until the others are in bed, then we will climb over the fence and get out of here. I've made reservations at a nearby hotel."

I don't think the breakout ever happened. They probably all forgot about it five minutes later. I admire their spirit.

MARCH 1, 2000

FINAL MOVE

I continue to visit Mom, even though we no longer have outings. They are too stressful for both of us, so I drop by to say hello. She has withdrawn again, so there is no longer any gossip about the locals. There are no longer any laughs or smiles. Really, there is nothing. She is vacant. It leaves my heart vacant. Her time on Earth is drawing to a close.

Last night, when I arrived, the administrator pulled me aside.

"Your mom has deteriorated rapidly over the past two days. She does not eat and will not get out of bed. Her bodily functions are shutting down. I'm afraid she needs to be moved to a higher level of care, where they can start hospice."

My mind was reeling. Was she really talking to me? It didn't seem real.

"Hospice," I thought. "It means …" I couldn't finish the thought. I didn't want to finish the thought. Everyone knows what hospice care means – there is no longer hope.

She recommended a convalescent hospital in El Cajon and said she would make all the arrangements. She told me they would move her for me.

I gave her the OK, and then I came home and cried myself to sleep. Today, I visited the convalescent hospital. The staff was caring, and the place was clean. It is in the city where I work. But ... the halls and rooms are filled by listless, groaning shells of what were once vibrant human beings. This is where people come to die. I researched the internet, and this place receives good marks. What choice do I have? I will cry myself to sleep again tonight.

MARCH 3, 2000

THE LAST CONVERSATION

Mom moves to the convalescent hospital tomorrow. I let the rest of the family know about the move. Things are moving faster than I thought they would.

I visited with her after work. I managed to get her out of bed and into her chair. I sat on the floor beside her and held her hand. She sat listlessly, but she was listening as I talked. She seemed to understand before the words were spoken.

I told her I loved her. I told her about moving to a hospital. I told her about my day. I rambled on and on. I wanted to make it as normal as could be.

She didn't say a word. She stared ahead, a vacant shell. Or, so it seemed. But when I kissed her goodbye and gave her a hug, I could feel her hug back. It was the first such returned contact in a very long time.

I hope hospice care can be arranged so she can come home for her last days or weeks. This is what end stage Alzheimer's does. It all really just sucks.

MARCH 6, 2000

IT'S TIME

I visit Mom in the convalescent hospital after work and on my lunch break each day. She is in a room by herself. I never stay long. I can't. I just cannot. It's hard seeing her there.

It's hard seeing all the sad, lonely souls there, watching the door as each visitor crosses the threshold of their Hell. Each aged face fills with hope that this visitor will be for them. Each aged face falls in disappointment when I walk by them to Mom's room. I try to smile and give them a kind "hello."

I keep hearing Dad angrily accusing me.

"I knew you God damned kids would lock us away in a rest home and forget us."

I hope he can see that I have not forgotten Mom. I am doing my best and doing what is best for her. I vow that I will never place such guilt on my children. I must ensure they know that I want them to do the same for me. They must not try to take on such a burden.

Mom's nurse told me today that hospice was notified and would be contacting me for hospice care arrangements. It's time, they told me. I need to bring her home to die.

MARCH 7, 2000

GOD SPEAKS

"How is your Mom?" the owner of the deli inquires, as I order a snack for my break. When you work in the field, you have your favorite stops, and this one on the east side of the city is one of mine. The owner has been following the current happenings in my life.

"I had to move her to a convalescent hospital here in town … ." I stop mid-sentence.

Was that a voice? Was that a thought? Was that a feeling? I don't know. All I know is I need to go to the hospital, now. My rational mind tells me, just wait for lunchtime. It has been my habit, now, to have lunch at Mom's side. But something else tells me to go.

"Judy, go now."

Who is that nagging me?

I feel a great urgency as I interrupt my conversation and head to my car. I speed through town to the west side. I am shaking, but why?

"Oh, thank goodness, you are here," a nurse tells me as I walk in the door. "We were just going to call you and tell you to come. Your mom has had a bad morning, and we don't think she will make it through the day."

I enter the room. "Is she sleeping or …?" I can see a slight rise and fall of her chest. I hear the sound of shallow breathing. She is still with us. My parents both had living wills, expressing in no uncertain terms that "heroic measures not be taken to save their lives."

I stand by the bed watching her. I take her hand and stroke her hair. She does not open her eyes, but I think I feel her squeeze ever so slightly.

"Mom, it's Judy. You've had such a rough time and fought so hard, but if you need to go now, it's OK. We will all be fine. You raised us to be strong and independent," I assure her.

She takes her last breath. As I hold her hand, I feel the life drain from her. I've heard when you are with someone who dies, you feel them go through you. I am not feeling that, but I am feeling her grateful sigh of release.

For some reason, I turn and look toward the far corner of the room. I don't see anything there, but I sense her presence.

"Go Mom. Be free. Have fun. I love you."

I say a short prayer: "Thank you God, for nagging me to 'go now'."

MARCH 14, 2000

PEACE FOR MOM, UNREST HERE

Family and friends gathered today in the tiny Alpine Baptist church for Mom's services, followed by burial at the Alpine Cemetery next to Dad. She died March 7, one month shy of her 84th birthday and one year and one month after Dad's death.

At her viewing, family members placed special mementos in the casket. Among them was the latest General Election ballot, placed there by her granddaughter, Kym. It was a fitting tribute for a woman who spent a lifetime politically fighting injustice, and serving in many political roles, including treasurer of the San Diego County Democratic Central Committee. She would have approved of this gesture.

Others "honored" her memory by making a quick trip to hers and Dad's attorney, two days after her death, and before the service arrangements were completed, to inquire about the estate, and their inheritance. Thankfully, the attorney shooed them out of the office, then called me.

Speakers at the funeral service recalled many warm and funny moments with Mom. One speaker misspoke while recalling Mom's bareback ride in cutoff jeans down Main Street of her small conservative Midwest town.

"Velva and a friend raised eyebrows when she and a friend rode, without clothes, on a horse down Main Street," he said, not catching the faux pas.

Now that would have really raised eyebrows, just as it raised a few snickers from guests at the service.

I am sure I heard her laughing from Heaven.

I hosted a memorial gathering at the house after the burial to honor hers and Dad's lives. Because of Mom's Alzheimer's, I was unable to do so after Dad's funeral. Sadly, some family members take to drinking on days like this, and some of my family members did just that and more. They left early, and I felt no sadness about that.

In fact, I have felt no sadness about Mom's death. Hers was a nearly two-decade long plunge into Alzheimer's Hell. I already grieved losing Mom about five years ago as she entered later stages of this horrible disease that steals the very essence of who you are. Death set her free. She was again Velva Dunbar, that restless soul always pulling at a society that binds women's freedom and muzzles their voices.

JANUARY 2013

EPILOGUE

Mom's story ended March 2000 when her soul left her fragile, Alzheimer's ravaged body. Since then, my life has had mostly ups, but lately it is heading downward. At 65, I worry that I am beginning to exhibit signs of the disease.

I expressed concern to my doctors, who assured me I don't have Alzheimer's. Just normal aging, they say. But they've never done any kind of screening. Never asked me one thing about why I think I'm in the early phase. One told me not to worry about it, just live each day that I have because there isn't anything I can do about it anyway.

There is a lot of flippancy in the medical community about this terminal disease – this disease that kills your soul, then your body. That is unsettling considering it affects an estimated 5.1 million Americans, according to the Alzheimer's Foundation of America. More, if you count the family members who watch their loved ones slowly fade into anonymity of Alzheimer's disease.

Alzheimer's is among the top 10 causes of death in the United States, and it is the only cause that cannot be cured or treated, according to the Alzheimer's Association. The rate of women with Alzheimer's outpaces that of men. Another American develops Alzheimer's disease every 68 seconds, Association literature states. The life expectancy of someone with Alzheimer's is from 2 years to 20 years, according to both organizations.

Studies have found some Alzheimer's genes that may increase a person's chance of contracting the disease.

In my family, we have lost not only my Mom, but two aunts and my grandmother to dementia. These weren't fast moving dementia cases. These women were robbed slowly and mercilessly of themselves for years before they died.

As for me, I sometimes feel dementia's insidious grip closing around my brain. I think I see the signs. I've always been a little scattered brained, unable to remember people's names and misplacing things. But, lately ... lately, this has been exacerbated. The signs are ominous. My vocabulary, which is extensive, is slipping away fast. I find myself struggling to pull the most common of words from my brain during conversations or even in my writings. After a two-year lay-off, I finally got temporary work. It was extremely hard for me to learn the simple job of a cashier at a register that does most of the work for you.

I use the wrong words for things – words that aren't even close to the subject. I will think the correct word, but say or write something completely out of context.

Learning, which once came easily, is now a struggle. Time gaps have become frequent. I don't know where I was during those gaps. I have no conscious memory of them. I just know I wasn't there.

My Uncle Roy tried to calm my fears by divulging that the family members who contracted Alzheimer's or dementia were also addicted to countless prescriptions drugs. At one time, when Mom was in the early stages, I counted 22 prescription medications to be taken at least once a day. How does one acquire so many prescriptions? Some play musical doctors, obtaining prescriptions from many different sources. Others, like Mom, manage to find one doctor unethical enough to prescribe them all.

I laugh off my Alzheimer's fears, as do my children, joking when I forget something. My children don't want to see it. Neither do I, but I must acknowledge the possibility. If I don't, no one will be ready when I lose myself.

My daughter Samantha, perhaps, sees it more than any other family member. We own a house together, so we are under one roof. She has seen my memory fade; she has seen me lose myself in those time gaps, and she has seen my increasing clumsiness such as when I fell off my low-heeled shoes, splat, on the ground. She admonishes me now if I wear anything other than flats.

She has not seen it all, however. I once fell on the stairway landing. Fortunately, I fell upward. If I had fallen the other way, I would have fallen all the way down the stairs. There was no reason. No tripping. I just fell. Some of the clumsiness may be due to my facial spasm medicine. It's as if my brain disconnects and doesn't give my body the signals it needs to function, much like what happens in Alzheimer's victims.

Samantha thinks I'm losing my hearing, but I'm not – recent hearing tests have proven only minor hearing loss in one ear. What I am losing is my ability to connect what is said to what my brain digests.

Sometimes I will be watching TV, and I can hear the words clearly, but can't comprehend what is said. The words sound like gibberish or a foreign language. Along this same line, I will sometimes be talking and the words start tripping out in speech patterns similar to a deaf person. At least that's how they sound to my ear. It's as if my mouth forgets how to form the words.

I also find myself doing things I would never do in the past. I am a fanatic about closing the cupboard doors and drawers – just ask my kids about my nagging them -- yet now I frequently find the doors and drawers standing wide open after I have been in the kitchen. I do not recall leaving them that way. With no one else home, I could be the only culprit. I've put things that belong in the fridge into the microwave and vice versa.

My thoughts derail during conversations. I find myself interrupting and speaking quickly for fear I will forget what I have to say – or even what the conversation was. When I try to explain something, I sometimes am unable to put the right words together, so I just ramble.

I think my kids are in denial. I understand that. I was once in their position. They, too, watched their grandmother slowly slip away for 20 years. I'm sure they don't want to watch the same thing happen to their mom.

But they need to be prepared. And they need to know they should feel no guilt if they must put me in a care facility. It is one thing to say you will take care of someone. It is a completely different story when you try to do it. I will not put that on my children. I only pray that they will be more patient and caring than I was with my own mother.

There is no happy ending to any story about Alzheimer's disease. Despite the hardships of caregiving, however, I would not exchange that last year I had with Mom for anything. It truly was a blessing. So maybe that is the happy ending.

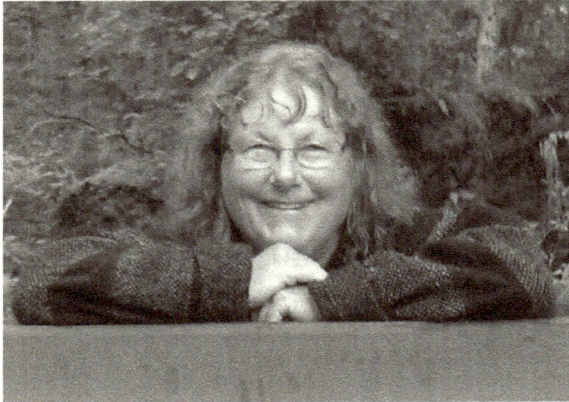

ABOUT THE AUTHOR

Judy Jones is a retired award-winning newspaper journalist, who lives in Southern California. She not only worked on civilian weekly and daily newspapers, but was managing editor of the Camp Pendleton Scout for eight years. She wasn't a Marine, but the Marines she worked with did and, still do, treat her like part of their family. Concurrent with her journalism career, she served for 20 years as a reserve deputy sheriff with the San Diego County Sheriff's Department both as a Search and Rescue Division deputy and a Law Enforcement Division deputy.

Leaving journalism to care for her mother, she eventually went to work for the City of El Cajon Police Department then moved to the City of Corona Building Department. Forced into early retirement by the economy, she has since taken seasonal jobs in Yellowstone and Olympic and National Parks in various positions. While working for park concessionaires, she volunteers for the National Park Service. Prior to this book, she wrote *Times Like These Vol. 1 … Christmas*, a memoir of Christmas joy, laughter and tears in the Jones family. *If I Forget, A Caregiver's Memories* started as the second in this series of books about post WWII family life, but has turned into so much more.

Ravages

(For Grandma Dunbar)
The ravages of age failed to erase
The beauty and gentleness in her sweet face.

When last I saw her, she laid shackled to bed.
By dementia's chains, she was bound.
Was that a flicker of knowing in her sad eyes?
Or was this grandchild just a face, a sound?

The ravages of age failed to erase
The beauty and gentleness in her sweet face.

Her hair she had pulled from her head;
Skin picked raw with fingers no longer nimble.
I closed my eyes so I could remember,
When her frail body did not so tremble.

The ravages of age failed to erase
The beauty and gentleness in her sweet face.

She stretched frail arms and nodded her head,
Toward the tiny bundle close to my breast.
She smiled; a tear slipped down her cheek,
As in her arms I laid my infant son at rest.

The ravages of age failed to erase
The beauty and gentleness in her sweet face.
Judy Jones

www.ingramcontent.com/pod-product-compliance
Lightning Source LLC
Chambersburg PA
CBHW022110280326
41933CB00007B/322